C000204723

BLUEPRINTS
Q&A Step 3
Obstetrics & Gynecology

Second Edition

BLUEPRINTS
Q&A Step 3
Obstetrics & Gynecology

Second Edition

Aaron B. Caughey, MD, MPP, MPH
Assistant Professor, Division of Maternal-Fetal Medicine
Department of Obstetrics & Gynecology
University of California, San Francisco
Division of Health Services and Policy Analysis
University of California, Berkeley
Berkeley & San Francisco, California

Deirdre J. Lyell, MD
Assistant Professor, Obstetrics & Gynecology
Stanford University School of Medicine
Attending Physician
Stanford University Medical Center
Stanford, California

Susan H. Tran, MD
Resident Physician, Obstetrics & Gynecology
Kaiser San Francisco Hospital
San Francisco, California

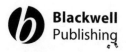

Blackwell
Publishing

Blackwell Publishing, Inc., 350 Main Street, Malden, Massachusetts 02148-5018, USA
Blackwell Publishing Ltd, 9600 Garsington Road, Oxford OX4 2DQ, UK
Blackwell Publishing Asia Pty Ltd, 550 Swanston Street, Carlton, Victoria 3053, Australia

04 05 06 07 5 4 3 2 1

ISBN: 1-4051-0395-7

Library of Congress Cataloging-in-Publication Data

Caughey, Aaron B.
    Blueprints Q&A Step 3. Obstetrics & gynecology / Aaron B. Caughey, Deirdre J. Lyell,
Susan H. Tran.—2nd ed.
        p. ; cm.—(Blueprints Q&A Step 3 series)
    Includes index.
    ISBN 1-4051-0395-7 (pbk.)
        1. Obstetrics—Examinations, questions, etc.   2. Gynecology—Examinations,
questions, etc.   3. Physicians—Licenses—United States—Examinations—Study guides.
    [DNLM: 1. Genital Diseases, Female—Examination Questions.   2. Delivery,
Obstetric—Examination Questions.   3. Pregnancy Complications—Examination Questions.
WP 18.2 C371b 2005]   I. Title: Blueprints Q&A Step 3. Obstetrics and gynecology.   II. Title:
Obstetrics & gynecology.   III. Lyell, Deirdre J.   IV. Tran, Susan H. V. Title.   VI. Series.
    RG111.C38 2005
    618′.076—dc22

                                                                    2004012942

A catalogue record for this title is available from the British Library

Acquisitions: Nancy Anastasi Duffy
Development: Kate Heinle
Production: Debra Murphy
Cover design: Hannus Design Associates
Interior design: Mary McKeon
Typesetter: Techbooks in New Delhi, India
Printed and bound by Capital City Press in Berlin, VT

For further information on Blackwell Publishing, visit our website:
www.blackwellmedstudent.com

Notice: The indications and dosages of all drugs in this book have
been recommended in the medical literature and conform to the practices of
the general community. The medications described do not necessarily have
specific approval by the Food and Drug Administration for use in the
diseases and dosages for which they are recommended. The package insert for
each drug should be consulted for use and dosage as approved by the FDA.
Because standards for usage change, it is advisable to keep abreast of
revised recommendations, particularly those concerning new drugs.

The publisher's policy is to use permanent paper from mills that operate a
sustainable forestry policy, and which has been manufactured from pulp
processed using acid-free and elementary chlorine-free practices. Furthermore,
the publisher ensures that the text paper and cover board used have met acceptable
environmental accreditation standards.

Contents

Contributors

Ryan Bradley
Class of 2004
University of California, San Francisco Medical School
San Francisco, California

Kimberly A. Gibson, MD, MPH
Resident, Department of Obstetrics & Gynecology
Kaiser Permanente, San Francisco
San Francisco, California

M. Rosanna Gray-Swain, MD
Resident, Department of Obstetrics & Gynecology
Washington University
St. Louis, Missouri

Amy E. Helmer, BA
Class of 2004
University of California, San Francisco Medical School
San Francisco, California

Mukesh Sahu
Class of 2004
University of California, San Francisco Medical School
San Francisco, California

Brian L. Shaffer, MD
Resident, Department of Obstetrics & Gynecology
University of California, San Francisco
San Francisco, California

Lishiana Solano-Shaffer, MD
Resident, Department of Obstetrics & Gynecology
Kaiser Permanente, Oakland
Oakland, California

Reviewers

Yessenia E. Coello, MD
PGY-1 Resident
New York Medical College
Valhalla, New York
Capitol Health Hospital
Trenton, New Jersey

Amanda Hallberg, MD
Family Medicine Resident
University of Michigan
Ann Arbor, Michigan

Vicki M. Trevino
Class of 2004
Samuel Merritt College Physician Assistant Program
Oakland, California

Preface

Thank you! We know that you, our customers, have successfully used the first edition of the Blueprints Q&A series to study for Boards and shelf exams. We also learned that those of you in physician assistant, nurse practitioner, and osteopath programs have found the series helpful to review for Boards and rotation exams.

At Blackwell, we think of our customers as our secret weapon. For every book Blackwell publishes, we rely heavily on the opinions of our customers, and we credit much of our success to the feedback we get from you. Your comments, suggestions—even complaints—help determine everything from content to features to the design of our books. The second edition of the Blueprints Q&A series is an excellent example of how much influence your feedback truly has:

○ You asked for more questions per book, so the questions have doubled (200 per book!).
○ You wanted questions that better reflect the format of the Boards, so all questions have been updated to match the current USMLE format for Step 3.
○ You liked the detailed explanations for every answer—right or wrong—so we made sure that complete correct and incorrect answers were provided for each question.
○ You needed a smaller trim size for easier portability, and now you have it. This edition is small enough to fit in a white coat pocket.
○ You were looking for an easier way to test yourself, and we redesigned this edition to do just that. Answer keys and tabbed sections make for easier navigation between questions and answers.
○ You wanted on index for easy reference, and you got it (along with abbreviations and normal lab values).

We hope you like this new edition of the Blueprints Q&A series as much as we do. And keep your suggestions and ideas coming! Please send any comments you may have about this book, or any book in the Blueprints series, to *blue@bos.blackwellpublishing.com*.

The Publisher
Blackwell Publishing

Acknowledgments

We would all like to thank the staff at Blackwell Publishing—particularly Kate Heinle and Nancy Duffy—for involving us in this project. I would also like to acknowledge my colleagues, whose support makes my work possible: the residents and faculty in the Departments of Obstetrics & Gynecology at the University of California, San Francisco, and the Brigham and Women's Hospital, Peter Callen, Mary Norton, and Gene Washington. I also thank my mother, father, Ethan, Samara, Big and Mugsy, and my new family—Ngan, Lieu, Mike, Vivian, Rob, Kim, Mike and Nancy, and Mamy, whose unflagging support during all of my projects keeps me on task and productive. This book is dedicated to The Bun and his college education.

—Aaron B. Caughey

This project is dedicated to the medical students, residents, faculty, and staff at Stanford Medical Center and the Brigham and Women's Hospital, and most of all to Jacob, Isabel, and Max.

—Deirdre J. Lyell

I would like to thank my friends and family for their support and encouragement. In particular, Mom and Dad, Mommaroonie and Pops, Mike and Viv, the girls, Rob and Rosaline, Kim and Mike, Nancy, Ethan, Samara, Soyoung and Cameron, Donna and Doug, Linda, Tina, Patricia, the Bhirridge, the Kaiser SF residents and staff, and, of course, my guys, Pi and The Bun, who make the journey meaningful.

—Susan H. Tran

Abbreviations

3TC	lamivudine (Combivir® or Trizivir®)	CMV	cytomegalovirus
5-FU	5-fluorouracil	CNS	central nervous system
17-OH	17-hydroxy	CPC	choroid plexus cyst
ABG	arterial blood gas	CPK	creatine phosphokinase
AC	abdominal circumference	CPR	cardiopulmonary resuscitation
ACE	angiotensin-converting enzyme	Cr	creatinine
ACTH	adrenocorticotropic hormone	CSF	cerebrospinal fluid
AF/AV	anteflexed, anteverted	CST	contraction stress test
AFI	amniotic fluid index	CT	computed tomography (CAT scan)
AFP	alpha-fetoprotein	CVA	cerebrovascular accident
AGA	appropriate for gestational age infant	CVAT	costovertebral angle tenderness
All	allergies	CVS	chorionic villus sampling
ALT	alanine transaminase	CXR	chest X-ray
AMA	advanced maternal age	D&C	dilation and curettage
ANA	anti-nuclear antibody	DCIS	ductal carcinoma in situ
ARDS	adult respiratory distress syndrome	D&E	dilation and evacuation
AROM	artificial rupture of membranes	DES	diethylstilbestrol
		DEXA	dual-energy X-ray absorptiometry
AST	aspartate transaminase	DHEA	dehydroepiandrosterone
AV	arteriovenous	DHEAS	dehydroepiandrosterone sulfate
AZT	zidovudine	DHT	dihydrotestosterone
BID	twice a day	DIC	disseminated intravascular coagulation
BP	blood pressure	DM	diabetes mellitus
BPD	biparietal diameter	DTR	deep tendon reflex
BPP	biophysical profile	DUB	dysfunctional uterine bleeding
β-hCG	beta human chorionic gonadotropin	DVT	deep vein thrombosis
		EBL	estimated blood loss
BTL	bilateral tubal ligation	ECC	endocervical curettage
BUN	blood urea nitrogen	ECG	electrocardiogram
BV	bacterial vaginosis	ED	emergency department
CAH	congenital adrenal hyperplasia	EDC	estimated date of confinement
CBC	complete blood count	EGA	estimated gestational age
CDC	Centers for Disease Control and Prevention	ELISA	enzyme-linked immunosorbent assay
CHOP	cyclophosphamide/doxorubicin/ oncovin/prednisone	EMBx	endometrial biopsy
		ESR	erythrocyte sedimentation rate
CIN	cervical intraepithelial neoplasia	ESWL	extracorporeal shock wave lithotripsy
CKC	cold knife cone	EtOH	ethanol, alcohol
CMF	cyclophosphamide/methotrexate/ 5-fluorouracil	FHR	fetal heart rate
		FHT	fetal heart tracing

FIGO	International Federation of Gynecology and Obstetrics		LDH	lactate dehydrogenase
FL	femur length		LEEP	loop electrosurgical excision procedure
FLM	fetal lung maturity		LFTs	liver function tests
FSH	follicle-stimulating hormone		LGA	large for gestational age infant
FTA-ABS	fluorescent treponemal antibody absorption		LGV	lymphogranuloma venereum
G	gravida		LH	luteinizing hormone
GA	gestational age		LMP	last menstrual period
GBS	Group B *Streptococcus*		LMW	low molecular weight
GC	gonococcal		LOC	loss of consciousness
GD	gestational diabetes		LSC	lichen simplex chronicus
GFR	glomerular filtration rate		LSIL	low-grade squamous intraepithelial lesion
GIFT	gamete intra-fallopian tube transfer		LSO	left salpingo-oophorectomy
GLT	glucose load test		MCV	mean corpuscular volume
GnRH	gonadotropin-releasing hormone		MHA-TP	microhemagglutination assay for antibodies to *T. pallidum*
GTD	gestational trophoblastic disease		MOM	milk of magnesia
GTT	glucose tolerance test		MRI	magnetic resonance imaging
GU	genitourinary		MSAFP	maternal serum alpha-fetoprotein
HC	head circumference		NGT	nasogastric tube
HELLP	hemolysis, elevated liver enzymes, low platelets		NKDA	no known drug allergies
hCG	human chorionic gonadotropin		NPO	nil per os (nothing by mouth)
Hct	hematocrit		NSAID	nonsteroidal anti-inflammatory drug
HDL	high-density lipoprotein		NST	nonstress test
HIV	human immunodeficiency virus		NT	nontender
HPI	history of present illness		NTD	neural tube defect
HPL	human placental lactogen		OCPs	oral contraceptive pills
HPP	history of present pregnancy		OCT	oxytocin challenge test
HPV	human papillomavirus		OGTT	oral glucose tolerance test
HR	heart rate		OHSS	ovarian hyperstimulation
HRT	hormone replacement therapy		OR	operating room
HSG	hysterosalpingography		P	para
HSIL	high-grade squamous intraepithelial lesion		PCA	patient-controlled analgesia
			PCOD	polycystic ovarian disease
HSV	herpes simplex virus		PCOS	polycystic ovarian syndrome
HTN	hypertension		PCR	polymerase chain reaction
ICSI	intra-cytoplasmic sperm injection		PDA	patent ductus arteriosus
Ig	immunoglobulin		PE	physical exam/pulmonary embolus
IM	intramuscular		PFTs	pulmonary function tests
INR	international normalized ratio		PGE$_{1M}$	prostaglandin E$_{1M}$—Cytotec/ misoprostol
IUD	intrauterine device			
IUFD	intrauterine fetal demise		PGE$_2$	prostaglandin E$_2$
IUGR	intrauterine growth restriction		PGF$_{2\alpha}$	prostaglandin F$_2$-alpha
IUI	intrauterine insemination		PGynHx	past gynecologic history
IUP	intrauterine pregnancy		PID	pelvic inflammatory disease
IUPC	intrauterine pressure catheter		PMDD	premenstrual dysphoric disorder
IV	intravenous		PMHx	past medical history
IVDA	intravenous drug abuse		PO	per os (by mouth)
IVF	in vitro fertilization		POBHx	past obstetric history
IVP	intravenous pyelography		POCs	products of conception
KOH	potassium hydroxide		POF	primary ovarian failure
KUB	kidneys/ureter/bladder		PPD	purified protein derivative
LCIS	lobular carcinoma in situ			

PPROM	preterm premature rupture of membranes	TAB	therapeutic abortion
PR	per rectum	TAH-BSO	total abdominal hysterectomy and bilateral salpingo-oophorectomy
PRBC	packed red blood cells	TFTs	thyroid function tests
PROM	premature rupture of membranes	TID	three times per day
PRN	as necessary	TNM	tumor/node/metastasis
PSHx	past surgical history	TOA	tubo-ovarian abscess
PT	prothrombin time	Tob	tobacco
PTL	preterm labor	TOC	tubo-ovarian complex
PTT	partial thromboplastin time	TOL	trial of labor
QD	once per day	TPN	total parenteral nutrition
QID	four times per day	TRH	thyrotropin-releasing hormone
RBC	red blood cell	TSH	thyroid-stimulating hormone
RDS	respiratory distress syndrome	TSS	toxic shock syndrome
ROM	rupture of membranes	TSST	toxic shock syndrome toxin
RPL	recurrent pregnancy loss	TZ	transformation zone
RPR	rapid plasma reagin	UA	urinalysis
RR	respiratory rate	US	ultrasound
RSO	right salpingo-oophorectomy	UTI	urinary tract infection
RUQ	right upper quadrant	VAS	vibroacoustic stimulation
SAB	spontaneous abortion	VDRL	Venereal Disease Research Laboratory
SBO	small bowel obstruction		
SC	subcutaneous	VBAC	vaginal birth after cesarean
SCC	squamous cell carcinoma	V/Q	ventilation/perfusion
SCJ	squamocolumnar junction	VS	vital signs
SGA	small for gestational age infant	VSD	ventricular septal defect
SPA	salt-poor albumin	VZIG	varicella zoster immunoglobulin
SROM	spontaneous rupture of membranes	VZV	varicella zoster virus
		WBC	white blood cell
SSE	sterile speculum exam	XAFP	expanded alpha-fetoprotein
STD	sexually transmitted disease	XR	X-ray
SVE	sterile vaginal exam	ZDV	zidovudine

Normal Ranges of Laboratory Values

Blood, Plasma, Serum

Alanine aminotransferase (ALT, GPT at 30°C)	8–20 U/L
Amylase, serum	25–125 U/L
Aspartate aminotransferase (AST, GOT at 30°C)	8–20 U/L
Bilirubin, serum (adult) Total // Direct	0.1–1.0 mg/dL // 0.0–0.3 mg/dL
Calcium, serum (Ca^{2+})	8.4–10.2 mg/dL
Cholesterol, serum	Rec: < 200 mg/dL
Creatine kinase, serum	Female: 10–70 U/L
Creatinine, serum	0.6–1.2 mg/dL
Electrolytes, serum	
Sodium (Na^+)	136–145 mEq/L
Chloride (Cl^-)	95–105 mEq/L
Potassium (K^+)	3.5–5.0 mEq/L
Bicarbonate (HCO_3^-)	22–28 mEq/L
Magnesium (Mg^{2+})	1.5–2.0 mEq/L
Follicle-stimulating hormone, serum/plasma	Female: premenopause 4–30 mIU/mL
	midcycle peak 10–90 mIU/mL
	postmenopause 40–250 mIU/mL
Glucose, serum	Fasting: 70–110 mg/dL
	2-h postprandial: < 120 mg/dL
Lactate dehydrogenase, serum	45–90 U/L
Luteinizing hormone, serum/plasma	Female: follicular phase 5–30 mIU/mL
	midcycle 75–150 mIU/mL
	postmenopause 30–200 mIU/mL
Osmolality, serum	275–295 mOsmol/kg
Parathyroid hormone, serum, N-terminal	230–630 pg/mL
Phosphate (alkaline), serum (p-NPP at 30°C)	20–70 U/L
Phosphorus (inorganic), serum	3.0–4.5 mg/dL
Prolactin, serum (hPRL)	< 20 ng/mL
Proteins, serum	
Total (recumbent)	6.0–7.8 g/dL
Albumin	3.5–5.5 g/dL
Globulin	2.3–3.5 g/dL
Thyroid-stimulating hormone, serum or plasma	0.5–5.0 μU/mL
Thyroidal iodine (^{123}I) uptake	8–30% of administered dose/24 h
Thyroxine (T_4), serum	5–12 μg/dL
Urea nitrogen, serum (BUN)	7–18 mg/dL
Uric acid, serum	3.0–8.2 mg/dL

Hematologic

Erythrocyte count	Female: 3.5–5.5 million/ mm^3
Erythrocyte sedimentation rate (Westergren)	Female: 0–20 mm/h
Hematocrit	Female: 36–46%
Hemoglobin A_{1C}	$\leq 6\%$
Hemoglobin, blood	Female: 12.0–16.0 g/dL
Leukocyte count and differential	
Leukocyte count	4500–11,000/mm^3
Segmented neutrophils	54–62%
Bands	3–5%
Eosinophils	1–3%
Basophils	0–0.75%
Lymphocytes	25–33%
Monocytes	3–7%
Mean corpuscular volume	80–100 μm^3
Partial thromboplastin time (activated)	25–40 s
Platelet count	150,000–400,000/mm^3
Prothrombin time	11–15 s
Reticulocyte count	0.5–1.5% of red cells

Urine

Calcium	100–300 mg/24 h
Creatine clearance	Female: 88–128 mL/min
Osmolality	50–1400 mOsmol/kg
Proteins, total	<150 mg/24 h
Sodium	Varies with diet

Questions

Setting 1: Community-Based Health Center

You work at a community-based health facility where patients seeking both routine and urgent care are encountered. Many patients are members of low-income groups; many are ethnic minorities. Several industrial parks and local businesses send their employees to the health center for treatment of on-the-job injuries and employee health screening. There is a facility that provides X-ray films, but CT and MRI scans must be arranged at other facilities. Laboratory services are available.

> **The next two questions (items 1 and 2) correspond to the following vignette.**

A 33-year-old G_1P_0 woman is seen in clinic at 39 weeks GA. Her fundal height measures 36 cm. You send her for US, which shows an estimated fetal weight of 3500 g, an amniotic fluid index (AFI) of 3.0, and normal uterine artery Dopplers. An US done earlier in the pregnancy showed normal amniotic fluid volume.

1. What is the most appropriate next step?

    A. Induction of labor
    B. Cesarean delivery
    C. Bed rest
    D. Maternal hydration
    E. Repeat US in 1 week

2. Which of the following is a possible etiology of oligohydramnios?

    A. Tracheoesophageal fistula
    B. Rh alloimmunization
    C. Gestational diabetes
    D. Renal agenesis
    E. Fetal hydrops

End of set

---

3. A 20-year-old presents 3 weeks past her missed period. She had unprotected intercourse once with someone not well known to her. Her office urine pregnancy test is positive. The patient wishes to terminate her pregnancy. Which of the following statements is true regarding pregnancy termination?

    A. In 1972, maternal mortality from illegal abortions was 52%; in 1974 it was 6%
    B. General anesthesia is now the major cause of mortality from pregnancy termination
    C. A single induced abortion does not cause future pregnancy complications or sterility
    D. Cervical dilation in the second trimester cannot safely be achieved by using laminaria
    E. Surgical termination is associated with a greater blood loss than is medical termination

4. A 31-year-old G_1P_0 presents to clinic at 26 weeks GA complaining of decreased fetal movement for 3 days. She has no medical problems and her pregnancy has been uncomplicated. She had a normal Level I US at 20 weeks GA. The patient's BP is normal, and her fundal height measures 26 cm. You are unable to auscultate fetal heart tones with a Doptone. Office US confirms fetal demise. Your partner comes in to confirm your finding, which you then explain to the patient. Which of the following do you recommend to the patient?

    A. Induction of labor
    B. Formal US to confirm findings
    C. Expectant management and await spontaneous labor
    D. Cesarean delivery
    E. Amniocentesis

The next two questions (items 5 and 6) correspond to the following vignette.

A 35-year-old G_4P_3 presents to clinic at 33 weeks GA after being involved in a minor motor vehicle accident. While pulling into your parking lot, another car collided with her front passenger door. The patient was wearing a seat belt, which had been placed low and across her lap, under her pregnant abdomen. She estimates that the other car was driving 5 to 10 miles per hour and reports minor damage to her car. She is unsure whether she hit her abdomen, and complains of mild left abdominal and shoulder pain. Your exam is unremarkable.

5. What is the most appropriate next step?

    A. 4 hours of fetal monitoring
    B. Draw a hematocrit
    C. Discharge home with follow-up in 1 week
    D. Rupture membranes to check for abruption
    E. Instruct the patient to follow fetal kick counts

6. Which of the following is true regarding management of a patient with major trauma during pregnancy?

    A. US can identify the majority of abruptions
    B. Pregnant patients generally show signs of shock later than nonpregnant patients
    C. Any pregnant patient with loss of consciousness should undergo emergent cesarean delivery
    D. If CPR is necessary, it can be performed similar to nonpregnant patients regardless of the trimester of pregnancy
    E. Fetal injury from trauma is common

End of set

---

7. An 18-year-old G_1P_0 presents to clinic at 36 weeks GA complaining of copious watery vaginal discharge that has run down her legs for the past 24 hours. Which of the following is the initial step in her evaluation?

    A. Culture for chlamydia
    B. Urine stream assessment for chlamydia
    C. Speculum exam and nitrazine test
    D. Cultures for herpes
    E. Office US

8. A 26-year-old woman presents complaining of a painful swollen mass near her vagina. She noticed a small lump approximately 2 weeks ago. During the last 2 days, the lump has become exquisitely tender and has grown significantly larger. The patient also reports subjective fevers. She has noticed no drainage, is not sexually active, and denies chills, myalgias, or vaginal discharge. On exam, you find a 4-cm, erythematous, nondraining vulvar mass to the right side of the posterior fourchette (Figure 8). What is the next step in management?

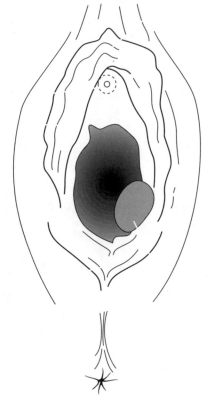

Figure 8 • Reproduced with permission from Callahan T. Blueprints Obstetrics & Gynecology. 3rd ed. Blackwell, 2004: Fig. 13-4, p. 126.

A. Oral antibiotics and follow-up in 1 week
B. Hospitalization and intravenous antibiotics
C. Full screen for sexually transmitted infections
D. Warm compresses
E. Incision and drainage

9. A 27-year-old G_0 presents with intermittent post-coital spotting for the past week. Her friend was recently diagnosed with cervical cancer, and the patient is extremely concerned that her bleeding is related to a similar diagnosis. She is sexually active with her husband only and has never had a sexually transmitted disease. She has had normal annual Pap smears for the past 5 to 6 years, with the most recent being 4 months ago. What is the most important initial diagnostic test?

    A. Pap smear
    B. Urine pregnancy test
    C. Chlamydia and gonorrhea culture
    D. Pelvic US
    E. Urine culture

10. A 47-year-old G_0 complains of moderate vaginal bleeding 3 weeks after her period, which lasted several hours, moderately stained two pads, and then stopped. She otherwise feels well, is non-obese, and is in good general health. Her menses are usually regular, occurring every 28 days and lasting for 3 to 4 days. Which of the following is the most important next step?

    A. Endometrial biopsy
    B. Pap smear
    C. Cervical cultures
    D. Pelvic US
    E. Hysteroscopy

11. A 39-year-old G_2P_0 presents after trying to become pregnant for 2 years. She is monogamous and sexually active with her husband twice a week. Her infertility evaluation has been normal, revealing normal cycles, normal thyroid and prolactin levels, and patent fallopian tubes. Her husband's semen analysis is normal. For the past one-and-a-half years, she has experienced increasingly heavy menstrual periods, and she has had two miscarriages. A pelvic US with injected saline is obtained (Figure 11). What is the most appropriate next step in management?

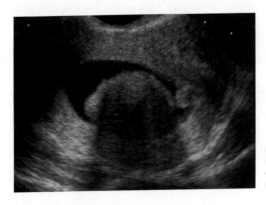

Figure 11 • Image provided by Departments of Radiology and Obstetrics & Gynecology, University of Calfornia, San Francisco.

    A. Adoption
    B. Recommend a gestational carrier
    C. Myomectomy
    D. Intra-cytoplasmic sperm injection (ICSI)
    E. In vitro fertilization (IVF)

12. A 27-year-old woman presents to the clinic reporting, "I have a skin rash down there." She believes the rash has been present for approximately 2 weeks. Other than a prior history of chlamydial infection at age 21, she denies any significant gynecologic or medical history. Which of the following is the most common noninfectious vulvar disease in members of this age group?

A. Eczema
B. Lichen simplex chronicus (LSC)
C. Lichen sclerosis
D. Melanoma
E. Basal cell carcinoma

13. A 36-year-old woman visits your clinic complaining of lesions on her labia. She denies any pain associated with the lesions, which appeared 3 days ago. She denies vaginal discharge, dysuria, or pruritis. On exam, you observe three 1-cm round, painless ulcers on her labia majora, and you note inguinal adenopathy. You suspect primary syphilis. Which of the following statements is true regarding this STD?

A. Early syphilis is treated with metronidazole for 14 days
B. Primary syphilis is characterized by a painless chancre that develops approximately 3 weeks after inoculation
C. The causative agent is a gram-positive rod
D. Secondary syphilis occurs when the lesions become painful and a rash appears on the backs of the hands and feet
E. Tertiary syphilis is characterized by notched teeth and saber shins

14. A 17-year-old G_1 student presents to the clinic for her second prenatal visit with uncertain GA. She was first seen 10 weeks ago, when she was unable to provide the date of her LMP, and was dated at 30 weeks by US (normal anatomy and amniotic fluid). Prenatal labs were drawn and were unremarkable except for an elevated 50-g glucose load test (GLT) of 163. The patient did not return for follow-up despite multiple messages being left by the clinic staff. She has never been counseled or treated for diabetes. This morning, she returns because she is extremely uncomfortable; however, she reports no symptoms of labor. She explains that she has not returned to clinic for fear of needing insulin injections like her mother and aunt, both of whom have diabetes. Her BP is 110/65. Urine dipstick shows 2+ glucose and trace protein. Her fingerstick blood glucose is 160, and the patient is certain that she has not eaten yet today. US estimates fetal weight at 5100 g, and fetal anatomy and amniotic fluid are normal. Fetal heart tracing is reactive. Which of the following diagnostic tests will be most useful in planning the obstetrical management of this patient?

A. Amniotic fluid lecithin:sphingomyelin ratio
B. 3-hour oral glucose tolerance test (OGTT)
C. Serum hemoglobin A_{1c} level
D. Cervical exam to assess Bishop score
E. Quantitative β-hCG

The following two questions (items 15 and 16) relate to the same clinical scenario.

A 28-year-old G_2P_1 woman at 32 weeks GA presents for a routine prenatal visit. Her previous pregnancy was uncomplicated, and she has had no problems in this pregnancy. Her BP in the office is noted to be elevated at 155/110, and her urine dips trace protein. She denies a prior history of hypertension. Her pressures have been normal earlier in this pregnancy. The patient does not complain of visual disturbances, headache, or epigastric discomfort. Her BPs are carefully monitored, and remain in the range 135–155/95–110. She is admitted to the hospital to rule out preeclampsia and to monitor her BPs. A 24-hour urine collection yields 160 mg of protein. The patient remains asymptomatic, and her pressures improve but remain elevated. The decision is made to discharge her to home with oral antihypertensive medication. She will monitor her BPs and urine protein at home.

15. Which of the following medications is the most appropriate choice in this setting?

   A. Labetolol
   B. Captopril
   C. Magnesium sulfate
   D. Losartan
   E. Furosemide

16. Over the next 4 weeks, the patient's BPs improve, and are generally in the range 110–125/80–95 with the use of her medication. Her urine occasionally dips trace proteinuria, but never higher. At 36 weeks GA, her membranes spontaneously rupture, and she delivers a healthy boy several hours later without complication. She now returns for her 6-week postpartum visit and brings a log of BPs, which are in the range 100–115/65–80. The patient explains that she is unsure what to tell friends and family about the reasons for her hospitalization during pregnancy. What is the most appropriate diagnosis of this patient's hypertension?

   A. Mild preeclampsia
   B. Severe preeclampsia
   C. Chronic hypertension
   D. Chronic hypertension with superimposed preeclampsia
   E. Gestational hypertension

End of set

17. A 38-year-old G_0 African American premenopausal woman presents to clinic for an annual exam. Her last exam was 3 years ago. She is 5 ft 7 in. tall and weighs 129 lb. Her physical exam is within normal limits except for the pelvic exam. On bimanual exam, you note a left adnexal mass, distinct from her uterus, which is retroverted and retroflexed. The mass is nontender and palpates approximately 6 to 7 cm in diameter. You order a pelvic US, which reveals an 8 cm × 7 cm × 5 cm complex left ovarian mass. No ascites or omental thickening is seen. The other ovary appears entirely normal. When considering how to counsel this patient about her differential diagnosis, which of the following statements is true regarding the major types of ovarian tumors?

   A. Epithelial cell tumors are the most common
   B. Epithelial cell tumors are more frequent among girls and young women
   C. Germ cell tumors include granulosa-theca and Sertoli-Leydig tumors
   D. Germ cell tumors are more frequent among women in their late fifties
   E. Sex-cord stromal tumors include mucinous and endometrioid tumors

---

The next two questions (items 18 and 19) correspond to the following vignette.

A mother brings her 15-year-old daughter to clinic, concerned because of the girl's abdominal pain. The pain began 2 months ago and has become constant. The patient is virginal and in good health. She has normal monthly menses and denies fevers, chills, nausea, vomiting, and weight loss. Pelvic US reveals a complex 8 × 6 cm left ovarian mass (Figure 18). The patient is taken to the operating room 2 days later for exploratory laparotomy and left salpingo-oophorectomy. The mass is removed without complication and sent to pathology for intraoperative frozen section analysis of tumor histology.

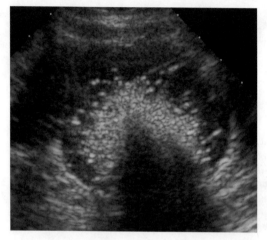

Figure 18 • Image provided by Department of Radiology and Obstetrics & Gynecology, University of California, San Francisco.

18. Which of the following associations is most accurate?

 A. Dysgerminoma arises from trophoblastic (placental) tissue
 B. Embryonal carcinoma arises from undifferentiated germ cells
 C. Endodermal sinus tumor arises from undifferentiated germ cells
 D. Choriocarcinoma arises from embryonic (fetal) tissue
 E. Immature teratoma arises from extraembryonic (yolk sac) tissue

19. Postoperative management of patients with ovarian tumors can include monitoring serum markers for evidence of persistent disease. Which of the following germ cell tumors is correctly matched to its associated serum tumor marker?

 A. Dysgerminoma and lactate dehydrogenase (LDH)
 B. Embryonal carcinoma and LDH
 C. Endodermal sinus tumor and CA-125
 D. Choriocarcinoma and alpha-fetoprotein (AFP)
 E. Immature teratoma and hCG

End of set

> **The next three questions (items 20, 21, and 22) correspond to the following vignette.**

A 29-year-old G_0 woman presents to the clinic with a nontender mass found on routine breast self-exam. Her family history is notable for breast cancer in an aunt at age 37. On physical exam, a firm, immobile mass is palpated in the upper outer quadrant of the left breast. No other masses are palpable, but axillary lymph nodes on the left side are firm and fixed. There is no discharge from the nipple. A bilateral mammogram is nondiagnostic (due to dense breast parenchyma). US identifies a 4-cm solid mass. MRI with contrast is consistent with infiltrating carcinoma. No involvement is seen on the right side, but several clinically occult lesions are apparent on the left side. Core biopsy of the 3-cm mass demonstrates histology consistent with medullary carcinoma, infiltrating the basement membrane. Tumor cells are found to be negative for estrogen receptors, progesterone receptors, and c-erbB-2 overexpression. Significant aneuploidy and a high S-phase fraction are seen. Axillary lymph node biopsy is positive for metastasis, but no other evidence of metastatic disease is noted on additional imaging or lab testing. The patient is determined to do everything possible to maximize her chances of curative therapy.

20. The planned surgical procedure will include resection of the breast tissue, nipple-areolar complex, overlying skin, and axillary lymph nodes. The pectoralis major muscle will be spared. What is the most accurate description of this procedure?

    A. Modified radical mastectomy
    B. Total (simple) mastectomy
    C. Subcutaneous mastectomy
    D. Radical mastectomy
    E. Wide local excision

21. Which of the following medical therapies would be most appropriate to start for this patient postoperatively?

    A. Hormonal therapy (e.g., tamoxifen)
    B. Combination chemotherapy (e.g., cyclophosphamide/methotrexate/5-fluoro-uracil, also known as CMF)
    C. Strontium-89
    D. Herceptin (trastuzumab)
    E. No therapy

22. Which of the following features of this patient's history and presentation has the most favorable impact on her prognosis?

    A. The tumor is negative for estrogen receptors
    B. The tumor is negative for progesterone receptors
    C. A high percentage of tumor cells is seen in the S phase
    D. The tumor is classified as medullary
    E. The patient is premenopausal

End of set

23. A 52-year-old G_0 woman presents to the clinic after a screening mammogram iden-tified a 3-cm lesion in the upper inner quadrant of her right breast. Physical exam is unremarkable, with no palpable breast masses. US-guided biopsy of the mass is positive for infiltrating intraductal carcinoma. A radionucleotide bone scan is negative for evi-dence of metastasis; chest and abdominal CT are unremarkable. A complete blood count and liver function tests are within normal limits. During surgery, the right axillary lymph nodes are noted to be firm, fixed, and positive for metastasis by intraoperative biopsy. No other evidence of metastasis is seen. Which of the following is the most accurate staging of this patient's disease?

A. Tis N0 M0 (Stage 0)
B. T1 N1 M0 (Stage IIa)
C. T3 N0 M0 (Stage IIb)
D. T2 N2 M0 (Stage IIIa)
E. T2 N2 M1 (Stage IV)

24. A 16-year-old African American woman presents to the clinic after 5 days of worsen-ing low abdominal pain. She reports nausea and vomiting, fever, and vaginal discharge. She is sexually active, currently has three partners, and is unsure of her LMP. She was seen in the ED 3 days ago and given "some pills," which she admits she did not take. On exam, she has uterine tenderness and pain with cervical motion. You note bilateral ad-nexal tenderness but cannot palpate her adnexa definitively. Her urine pregnancy test is negative. You diagnose PID. Which of the following is the best next step in management?

A. Transvaginal US to rule out tubo-ovarian abscess
B. Serum β-hCG since she is unsure of her LMP
C. Oral antibiotics with another clinic appointment within 24 hours
D. Admission for laparoscopy
E. Admission with intravenous antibiotics

25. A 36-year-old G_3P_3 presents to your clinic 8 days after an uncomplicated IUD insertion. She noted increasing pain and vaginal spotting. Her recent cervical cultures for gonorrhea and chlamydia were negative at the time of the IUD insertion, and she reports no intercourse with her husband in the last 5 weeks. She is afebrile but has uterine tenderness on bimanual exam. Which of the following is the best option for management?

A. Admission with intravenous antibiotics
B. Outpatient oral antibiotics
C. Removal of IUD and oral antibiotics
D. Repeat cultures and prescribe NSAIDs
E. Check a urine pregnancy test

26. A 27-year-old woman and her boyfriend of 8 months regularly engage in sexual relations using condoms as their sole form of birth control. They are careful and have never had a problem with breakage or slippage in the past. Two days after their last sexual encounter, however, the woman receives a call from her boyfriend, who states that the condom may have broken during sex. He had refrained from saying something sooner because he wasn't sure and did not want to worry her, but after giving the matter more thought now feels that the breakage did indeed occur. Fearing the worst, the woman considers using emergency contraception, or "the morning after pill," to prevent pregnancy. Which of the following statements is most accurate regarding the benefit of emergency contraception for this woman?

A. She will not benefit because the event occurred more than 24 hours prior to taking the pill

B. She may not benefit because the failure rate with emergency contraception approaches 25%

C. She may benefit depending on her ability to obtain a prescription from her gynecologist promptly

D. She may benefit as long as she is willing to accept the risk of teratogenicity to the fetus should the regimen fail

E. She may benefit because she has never used an IUD

27. A 32-year-old woman had a low-grade squamous intraepithelial lesion (LSIL) on her annual Pap smear. She underwent colposcopic evaluation. At the time of colposcopy, the transformation zone (TZ) was visible clockwise from 1 o'clock to 10 o'clock. Two areas of concern were biopsied. An endocervical curettage (ECC) was also done. The pathology from one biopsy was "Normal exocervix," and that from the other biopsy was "High-grade squamous intraepithelial lesion (HSIL). No evidence of invasion." The ECC pathology was negative. Which of the following options should this woman be offered?

A. Hysterectomy

B. Repeat colposcopy in 3 months

C. Loop electrosurgical excision procedure (LEEP)

D. Localized radiation therapy

E. Cryotherapy

28. A 32-year-old G_4P_3 woman presents at 19 weeks GA for a routine prenatal appointment immediately prior to her scheduled US. She has had an uncomplicated antenatal course with normal first-trimester labs. In addition, her triple screen returned negative for neural tube defects or aneuploidy. The patient and her husband are looking forward to the US because they have three daughters and are hoping for a son. You discuss the indications for a Level I obstetric US. Which of the following is a routine component of this US?

A. Fetal extremities

B. Fetal gender

C. Fetal kidneys

D. Umbilical cord insertion into the placenta

E. Fetal face

29. A 20-year-old G_1P_0 woman at 16 weeks GA by LMP has decided she wants to terminate the pregnancy. She is healthy and denies prior medical or surgical history. What is the safest and most appropriate method to induce an abortion in this patient?

A. Suction curettage

B. Vaginal prostaglandin administration

C. Menstrual regulation

D. Hysterectomy

E. D&E

30. A 37-year-old G_3P_3 woman asks you to discuss birth control options. She does not want to risk becoming pregnant again at her age, but feels that sterilization is "a bit drastic." She has a history of postpartum depression, no other past medical history, smokes one-half pack of cigarettes a day, and has no allergies to medications. What is the most efficacious method of contraception for this patient without any contraindications?

A. Depo-Provera
B. Combined OCPs
C. Progestin-only OCPs
D. Diaphragm
E. Copper-T IUD

31. A 16-year-old woman has just recently become sexually active and comes to your clinic for her first annual exam. At the end of the exam, she expresses interest in starting OCPs to prevent pregnancy while she finishes school. Her health counselor once told her, however, that some women should not take birth control pills because it could be hazardous to their health. She is concerned that she may be one of those women. To allay her concerns, you decide to take a more thorough history and highlight for her the factors that would be considered dangerous. Of the following, what additional history would be considered an absolute contraindication to combined OCPs?

A. History of diabetes mellitus type I
B. Concurrent hypertension (HTN)
C. Uterine leiomyoma (fibroid)
D. Family history of breast cancer
E. Concurrent symptomatic hepatitis C infection

32. A 35-year-old G_2P_1 woman presents to your clinic 4 weeks after spontaneous abortion of a highly desired pregnancy at 10 weeks GA. She reports 1 week of persistent, intermittent vaginal bleeding and 2 days of hemoptysis. Physical exam is notable for tachycardia and an enlarged uterus. Speculum exam reveals only a small amount of blood in the vaginal vault. A β-hCG level is drawn and is found to be elevated at 25,000 mIU/mL. Suction curettage is performed, and after pathology confirms the diagnosis, imaging is ordered. Multiple pulmonary nodules are identified on chest X-ray; chest CT confirms the nodules seen on plain film. CT of the abdomen and brain are within normal limits, with no focal lesions identified. What is the most appropriate medical treatment to initiate for this patient?

A. Single-agent chemotherapy (e.g., methotrexate)
B. Multiple-agent chemotherapy (e.g., etoposide/methotrexate/dactinomycin)
C. Hysterectomy
D. Exploratory laparotomy and local excision of uterine lesion
E. Radiation therapy to pelvis

33. A 24-year-old G_1P_0 woman—a patient of another physician in your practice who is currently on vacation—presents to your office 6 weeks after suction evacuation of an incomplete molar pregnancy. She was started on OCPs at that time, and has been compliant with her medication. Her β-hCG level today is 3000 mIU/mL, slightly lower than the value of 5000 mIU/mL measured last week. Today, the patient expresses her desire to conceive, and says that she does not understand why she needs to continue with contraceptives. What is the most compelling reason for her to continue taking the OCPs?

A. She is at increased risk for GTD in future pregnancies, and the risk is significant enough to discourage future pregnancy

B. She is at increased risk of spontaneous abortions, complications, and congenital malformations in future pregnancies, and these risks are significant enough to discourage future pregnancy

C. OCPs reduce the risk of persistent locally invasive moles

D. OCPs reduce the risk of malignant choriocarcinoma

E. Reliable prevention of pregnancy is necessary to allow accurate measurement of β-hCG levels to rule out persistent or malignant trophoblastic disease

34. A 39-year-old G_2P_0 presents for a routine office visit at 30 weeks GA. Her pregnancy has been unremarkable, and she has no history of medical problems or UTIs. Today in the clinic, her BP is 90/60. A routine urine dipstick reveals trace protein, trace blood, trace leukocyte esterase, and 1+ WBCs. She denies dysuria, fevers, chills, contractions, vaginal bleeding, and leakage of fluid, and reports good fetal movement. What is the most appropriate next step?

A. Send a urine culture

B. Counsel her to follow up if she becomes symptomatic

C. Treat with antibiotics

D. Do nothing

E. Renal biopsy

35. A 15-year-old G_1P_0 woman presents at 33 weeks GA complaining of constant abdominal pain for 2 days. She has been leaking fluid for approximately 1 week. She feels otherwise well and denies symptoms of an upper respiratory tract infection, nausea, vomiting, diarrhea, or dysuria. Her appetite is normal. On exam, she is febrile to 101.1°F, her pulse is 120, her abdomen is tender to palpation, and she has a foul-smelling, purulent vaginal discharge. There is no pool of fluid in her vagina, but a fern pattern is seen on a slide, and nitrazine paper turns dark blue when touched with the swab. The patient's cervix appears long and closed. Office US reveals a fetus in cephalic presentation and an amniotic fluid index of 2. What is the most appropriate next step?

A. Cesarean section

B. Antibiotics and observation

C. Amniocentesis for culture

D. Tampon dye test

E. Induction of labor

36. A 27-year-old G_3P_0 presents to clinic at 26 weeks GA complaining of constant vaginal wetness that began 3 weeks ago. She now wears a pad in her underwear because of her symptoms. She experiences occasional vaginal itching and mild pain. The patient has no medical problems, and her pregnancy has been uncomplicated. She denies contractions, vaginal bleeding, and abnormal discharge, and reports active fetal movement. What is the most important and appropriate next step in this patient's management?

A. Observation at home with further evaluation if the symptoms worsen

B. Sterile speculum exam with tests for a pool of fluid with a fern pattern and a basic pH

C. Sterile speculum exam with a KOH and wet prep

D. Vaginal and rectal swab for Group B *Streptococcus*

E. US

37. A 34-year-old G_3P_2 at 32 weeks GA calls your clinic concerned because her son's friend, who just slept overnight at their home, awoke with a vesicular rash, which has been confirmed to be chickenpox. The patient is unsure whether she has had chickenpox. She is feeling well and has no medical problems. Her pregnancy has been uncomplicated. You recommend that she do which of the following?

A. Go to the clinic for an exam
B. Go to the ED designated area for varicella zoster immunoglobulin (VZIG)
C. Go to the pharmacy and fill a prescription for oral acyclovir
D. Alert the pediatrician so that the infant may be prophylaxed after delivery
E. Go to the ED designated area and have a varicella zoster virus (VZV) titer drawn

38. A 20-year-old G_3P_0 presents at 16 weeks GA for her first prenatal visit. Her prenatal labs are normal except her RPR, which is reactive. She has no medical problems and takes no medications. She has had three sexual partners during the last year, has had sexual contact with two of the partners in the last 3 months, and has used condoms only occasionally. She had a full STD-screen 1 year ago, including an RPR, which was negative. She feels well in general, but during the last 6 months has experienced three episodes of arthritis of her hands, lasting approximately 2 weeks before resolving spontaneously. She reports intermittent fatigue during the last 2 years, which was not significant enough to prevent her from exercising but has worsened since she became pregnant. She denies fever, rash, and photosensitivity. What is the most appropriate next step?

A. Send an ANA
B. Arrange a consult with rheumatology
C. Send an MHA-TP
D. Treat with benzathine penicillin G
E. Repeat the RPR

39. A 37-year-old G_2P_1 Caucasian woman presents to you at 33 weeks GA with her third complaint of decreased fetal movement in the last 3 weeks. You send her for a nonstress test, which is reactive. She appears tremendously relieved. An amniocentesis at 16 weeks was normal, and US revealed an appropriately grown fetus without identifiable anomalies and a posterior placenta. Her fundal height measures appropriately. She is 5 ft 5 in. tall, weighs 140 lb, and has gained 12 lb during this pregnancy. She reports that poor appetite has been a problem, and she has been trying to increase her caloric intake. She is married, and describes her husband as somewhat ambivalent about the pregnancy because of financial concerns. During this pregnancy, she has come in nearly weekly complaining of any variety of mild symptoms, including headaches, abdominal pain, decreased fetal movement, joint pains, and heartburn, each time wanting reassurance that the baby is okay. She is well known to you because you delivered her first child, and she did not have multiple somatic complaints during that pregnancy. What is the most appropriate next step in this patient's management?

A. Biophysical profile
B. Screen for domestic violence
C. Evaluate for anorexia nervosa
D. US for fetal weight
E. Weekly nonstress tests

40. A mother brings her 16-year-old G_0 daughter to the clinic because she has not yet begun to menstruate. On exam, the girl is 5 ft 9 in. tall and weighs 100 lb. Her breasts are enlarged, and the areolae project to form secondary mounds. She shaves her axilla and has a mid-escutcheon on her mons. Her vagina appears well estrogenized, there is no septum, and her cervix appears normal. On palpation, a uterus is present, and her ovaries feel normal. Which Tanner stage of development (Figure 40a) best describes this patient?

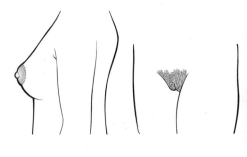

Figure 40a · Reproduced with permission from Callahan T. Blueprints Obstetrics & Gynecology. 3rd ed. Blackwell, 2004: Figs. 20-2 and 20-3, p. 181.

A. Stage 1
B. Stage 2
C. Stage 3
D. Stage 4
E. Stage 5

41. A 16-year-old adolescent female is brought in by her mother for what appears to be primary amenorrhea. Upon further questioning, she admits that she had her first period at age 14, had four periods every 1 to 2 months after that, and has not a period for more than 1 year. You ask her mother to leave the room. The patient reports that she has lost 20 lb during the last year and a half as a result of dieting and exercising 1 hour a day. Reluctantly, she admits that she feels fat, and she describes her friends as serial dieters. The patient does not like to discuss her weight with her mother, who has encouraged her to gain weight. She is 5 ft 9 in. tall and weighs 100 lb. Her exam is normal, and development is otherwise appropriate for her age. She has no medical problems, is virginal, and has never had surgery. A urine pregnancy test is negative. Which of the following is the most likely cause of this patient's secondary amenorrhea?

A. Cervical stenosis
B. Asherman's syndrome
C. Premature ovarian failure (POF)
D. Hypothalamic amenorrhea
E. Polycystic ovarian syndrome (PCOS)

42. A 21-year-old G_0 woman presents complaining of profuse, foul-smelling, greenish vaginal discharge, which worsened 2 days after the end of her LMP. She complains of itching and irritation. She is sexually active, has had two partners during the last 3 months, and does not use condoms. On sterile speculum, she has a frothy gray-green discharge. You perform a wet prep in clinic and see actively moving, flagellated organisms. Figure 42 shows a scanning electron micrograph of the organism. Which of the following statements is true regarding this patient?

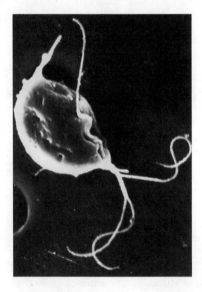

Figure 42 • Reproduced with permission from Cox FEG, ed. Modern Parasitology: A Textbook of Parasitology. 2nd ed. Blackwell Science, 1993: Fig. 9.

A. She can be treated immediately with 2 g of oral metronidazole (Flagyl)
B. Her partners do not need treatment, as men do not manifest symptoms of this infection
C. She can be treated with 250 mg of oral azithromycin (Zithromax)
D. There is no need to screen for STDs such as *Neisseria gonorrhea, Chlamydia trachomatis,* and HIV
E. Diagnosis cannot be made on wet prep alone; prior to treatment, a culture should be sent to confirm the diagnosis

43. A 22-year-old G_1P_1 woman complains of a foul-smelling vaginal discharge and dyspareunia for 3 days. She has been sexually active with her new partner for 1 month and uses oral contraception, but not condoms. She has had one other sexual partner during the last year and did not use condoms. Her LMP was 8 days ago. The patient is compliant and well known to you. On exam, she is afebrile. Her abdomen is nontender. Her pelvic exam is pertinent for mucopurulent discharge coming from her cervical os, cervical-motion tenderness, and a nontender uterus and adnexae. Which of the following is the most appropriate initial treatment?

A. Ceftriaxone 250 mg IM once
B. Ceftriaxone 250 mg IM once and azithromycin 1g PO once
C. Doxycycline 100 mg PO BID × 7 days
D. Azithromycin 1 g PO once
E. Cefoxitin 2 g IV q6 hours and doxycycline 100 mg IV q12 hours

44. A 48-year-old G_2P_2 woman presents with menorrhagia, bloating, and pelvic pressure. During the past 2 years, her menses have lasted longer and are heavier. She has also begun to experience dyspareunia and constipation. Rectovaginal exam is remarkable for fullness. Pelvic US reveals an 8 cm × 8 cm × 6 cm homogeneous fibroid in the posterior uterine wall. Which of the following statements is true about fibroids?

A. Most women with fibroids eventually become symptomatic
B. Fibroids should be removed because of their malignant potential
C. Fibroids tend to regress during pregnancy
D. Fibroids are associated with infertility
E. Fibroids are most common among Hispanic women

45. A 31-year-old G_0 woman is found to have moderate cervical intraepithelial neoplasia (CIN II) on her Pap smear. Colposcopically directed biopsies are consistent with CIN II at two small sites on the exocervix. The endocervical curettage (ECC) is normal. The patient has always had normal annual Pap smears, with the most recent occurring 1 year ago. She has had a new sexual partner for the last 6 months and uses oral contraception. What is the most appropriate next step in this patient's treatment?

A. Serotype for HPV
B. Cryotherapy or laser therapy
C. Loop electrosurgical excision procedure (LEEP)
D. Cold knife cone (CKC)
E. Repeat colposcopy and biopsies in 3 months

46. A 62-year-old G_2P_2 woman, postmenopausal for 12 years, presents to the clinic complaining of abdominal bloating for 6 months. During the past 2 months she has been unable to button her pants, despite a 10-lb weight loss achieved without dieting. A pelvic US reveals massive ascites and a 9 cm × 10 cm complex right ovarian mass (Figure 46). In addition to obtaining lab work, what is the next step in this patient's management?

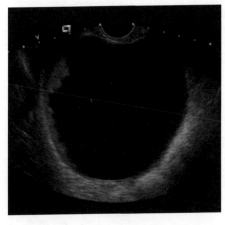

Figure 46 · Image provided by Departments of Radiology and Obstetrics & Gynecology, University of California, San Francisco.

A. Observation with repeat US in 4 weeks
B. Exploratory laparotomy
C. Diuretic treatment for relief of her ascites
D. A second opinion
E. Chemotherapy

47. A 24-year-old G_1P_0 woman at 18 4/7 weeks GA presents to the clinic after her scheduled US. The radiologist calls you to report an abnormality, which is shown in Figure 47. The patient had an expanded AFP (XAFP) serum screening test sent off 3 days ago as well, but the results are not back yet. Based on the findings in the US in Figure 47, what are the likely results of her XAFP?

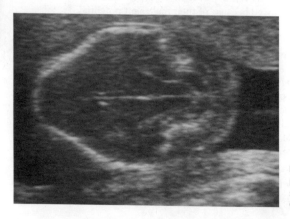

Figure 47 · Image provided by Departments of Radiology and Obstetrics & Gynecology, University of California, San Francisco.

A. Decreased MSAFP, decreased estriol, elevated hCG
B. Decreased MSAFP, decreased estriol, decreased hCG
C. Elevated MSAFP, normal estriol, normal hCG
D. Elevated MSAFP, elevated estriol, elevated hCG
E. Normal MSAFP, decreased estriol, elevated hCG

48. A 23-year-old G_0 woman presents with intermittent left lower quadrant pain. The pain began 2 months ago, a couple of weeks before her monthly menses. She describes the pain as mild, sharp, focal, nonradiating, and never severe. The patient is virginal and takes no medications. She is afebrile and well appearing. Pelvic exam reveals fullness in the left adnexa. A pelvic US demonstrates a 2-cm simple left adnexal cyst. What is the most appropriate next step?

A. Oral progestin-only pills
B. Laparoscopic cystectomy
C. Fine-needle aspiration
D. Hospitalization and observation
E. Outpatient observation

49. A 55-year-old woman comes to the clinic with complaints of a vulvar lesion for at least the past 6 months. The mass appears suspicious for malignancy, and you perform a vulvar biopsy, which returns as Paget's disease. Which of the following statements is true about Paget's disease of the vulva?

    A. Treatment is wide local excision or vulvectomy without radiation or chemotherapy

    B. It is caused by HPV

    C. It is associated with a lower incidence of an underlying internal carcinoma than other forms of Paget's disease

    D. It is most common in premenarchal females

    E. It is commonly associated with HSV-1

50. An 18-year-old African American woman presents to the clinic after 5 days of worsening lower abdominal pain. She reports nausea and vomiting, fever, and vaginal discharge. She is sexually active with three partners and is unsure of her LMP. She was seen in the ED 3 days ago and given "some pills," which she admits she did not take. On exam, she is afebrile and has uterine and cervical motion tenderness. You also note bilateral adnexal tenderness and no vaginal discharge. Her urine pregnancy test is negative. You diagnose pelvic inflammatory disease and emphasize the importance of taking the prescribed antibiotics. However, the patient returns 4 days later still complaining of pain. She now has a fever. An US reveals bilateral tubo-ovarian abscesses (TOAs). Which of the following statements is true regarding TOA?

    A. TOA results from a mixed polymicrobial infection with a high proportion of anaerobes

    B. Management should begin with drainage of the complex

    C. TOA is most commonly caused by appendicitis, pelvic surgery, or diverticulitis

    D. Fever and elevated WBC count are the most common features of TOA

    E. TOA is not associated with future infertility as compared to PID

Answers and Explanations

Answer Key

1. A		18. E		35. E	
2. D		19. A		36. B	
3. C		20. A		37. E	
4. A		21. B		38. C	
5. A		22. D		39. B	
6. B		23. D		40. D	
7. C		24. E		41. D	
8. E		25. C		42. A	
9. B		26. B		43. B	
10. A		27. C		44. D	
11. C		28. C		45. B	
12. B		29. E		46. B	
13. B		30. E		47. C	
14. A		31. E		48. E	
15. A		32. A		49. A	
16. E		33. E		50. A	
17. A		34. A			

1. **A.** An AFI of less than 5 cm is diagnostic of oligohydramnios. Late in pregnancy, unexplained oligohydramnios should prompt concern for placental insufficiency and nonreassuring fetal status. A stressed fetus shunts blood away from the kidneys and toward the brain, resulting in decreased renal perfusion, decreased urine production, and eventually oligohydramnios. A fetus with oligohydramnios at term should be delivered. Induction of labor is reasonable, although the fetus may not tolerate labor well.

   B. Cesarean delivery is not necessary based on the finding of oligohydramnios alone.

   C, D. Bed rest and maternal hydration are thought to improve uterine perfusion, which in turn may improve fetal perfusion and amniotic fluid volume. Oligohydramnios may indicate nonreassuring fetal status and should indicate prompt delivery at term. These options might be employed if the fetus is premature.

   E. Waiting 1 week is not appropriate. Antepartum fetal testing is performed to identify the fetus at risk for intrauterine fetal demise or abnormal outcome.

2. **D.** Amniotic fluid is produced primarily by the fetal kidneys and less by the fetal lungs. Thus renal agenesis leads to oligohydramnios or anhydramnios. Amniotic fluid provides an acoustic window for US, which is quite limited in the setting of anhydramnios or severe oligohydramnios. US with Doppler can be used to identify the renal arteries, which suggest the presence of kidneys. Absence of the renal arteries suggests absence of kidneys.

   A. From the second trimester onward, fetal swallowing and urination result in continuous circulation of amniotic fluid. Disorders of the gastrointestinal tract, such as tracheoesophageal fistula, generally result in polyhydramnios, not oligohydramnios.

   B, E. Rh alloimmunization (known also as isoimmunization) leads to fetal hemolysis, anemia, and eventually fetal hydrops. This results in polyhydramnios rather than oligohydramnios.

   C. Uncontrolled gestational diabetes can be associated with fetal macrosomia and polyhydramnios similar to pregestational diabetes.

3. **C.** Having one or more prior abortions is unlikely to be associated with an increased risk of adverse outcomes in subsequent pregnancies. A history of three or more induced abortions appears to be associated with pregnancy complications such as placental abruption, premature rupture of the membranes, low birth weight, preterm delivery, and bleeding in the first and third trimesters as compared to women with a history of two or fewer induced abortions.

   A. Illegal abortions resulted in significant maternal mortality (some studies reported rates as high as 39% prior to legalization of abortion), but the rate was not as high as 52%. A mere 2 years after the *Roe v. Wade* decision in 1972, maternal mortality fell dramatically to 6%, largely due to increased access to procedures performed sterilely in adequate medical facilities by trained, accountable practitioners. Today, maternal mortality is close to zero in the United States in patients with no medical complications who undergo routine procedures.

B. General anesthesia is rarely needed in pregnancy termination, except in cases of extreme anxiety, mental retardation, or psychotic disorders. While general anesthesia poses the greatest risk to a woman undergoing pregnancy termination, most such procedures are performed with the use of a paracervical block, often in combination with a sedative. Thus general anesthesia is not a major cause of mortality due to pregnancy termination.

D. Laminaria, often composed of hygroscopic seaweed, are placed into the cervix to facilitate cervical dilation prior to the procedure. The laminaria take on liquid, which results in their expansion and gentle dilation of the cervix. Gradual dilation reduces the risk of cervical trauma and is safe for usage in both first- and second-trimester terminations.

E. Medical termination is associated with more bleeding than surgical termination. However, overall blood loss from both procedures is low.

4.
> **A.** Upon the diagnosis of intrauterine fetal demise (IUFD), immediate delivery is offered. Case reports do cite maternal coagulopathy developing in association with IUFD, but this complication has been shown to occur only when the IUFD took place 3 weeks or more beforehand. Many patients with IUFD may want to delay delivery for a few days to grieve prior to undergoing the stress of labor. As long as the risk of coagulopathy is explained to the patient and screened for, this is reasonable management. Occasionally, patients will not want to go through labor with an IUFD and will request a cesarean delivery. Because of the risks to the patient from cesarean delivery as well as its effects on all future pregnancies, this is not a reasonable course of action. Patients and their partners should be encouraged to name, hold, and view the demised fetus. At the time of delivery, a nurse or assistant may take the stillborn to another room to examine it and describe it to the family, especially if the stillborn is macerated or anomalous. He or she should then swaddle and place a hat on the stillborn, like a newborn, and, if the parents have agreed, bring it to them. Viewing, holding, and naming the baby have been shown to facilitate the grieving process. In the case of anomalous or macerated fetuses, studies have shown that the actual experience of viewing the baby is better than the nightmarish fantasies that people may otherwise have.

B. Fetal demise should be confirmed by a second person skilled in US. Both examiners should observe absence of fetal cardiac activity for at least 3 minutes. You appropriately asked your partner to confirm the diagnosis. A third US is not necessary. Note that if the patient had not had an US performed for anatomy, it would not be unreasonable to obtain an US to look for an anatomic cause for fetal demise (e.g., congenital abnormality or syndrome). However, the best way to identify such an etiology is with post-delivery exam by pathology.

C, D. See the explanation for A.

E. Amniocentesis may be performed most commonly in the second trimester for prenatal diagnosis to obtain fetal cells to perform a karyotype or other genetic tests. It is also performed later in pregnancy to assess fetal lung maturity. There would be no reason to obtain these tests at this point. However, a karyotype would be one aspect of the postpartum work-up of the IUFD.

5. | **A.** The incidence of perinatal mortality following minor trauma is 0.5%. Thus all seemingly minor traumas must be evaluated. The standard of care is to assess the fetal heart rate and tocometer for 4 to 6 hours following trauma, looking for contractions that may not be apparent to the patient and performing fetal evaluation. Monitoring should be extended, with consideration for delivery, if the fetal testing is nonreassuring, there are signs of placental abruption, or the trauma is significant.

B. A hematocrit will not be helpful in guiding management after this minor trauma. A Kleihauer-Betke test may be used to screen for fetal–maternal hemorrhage due to placental abruption. Pregnant women generally have a physiologic anemia, and a single hematocrit is not useful. In cases of severe trauma, serial hematocrits may be appropriate.

C. Placental abruption may develop over hours or even a couple of days. Thus, if the patient is discharged home after 4 hours of fetal monitoring, she should be advised to follow up for any symptoms of uterine contractions, abdominal pain, or decreased fetal movement. Before discharge home, however, the patient should be monitored as in the explanation for A.

D. If the patient was full term and her cervix was favorable, one could consider induction of labor after minor trauma, particularly if monitoring was nonreassuring. Rupture of membranes, when appropriate during induction, might reveal blood-tinged amniotic fluid following trauma. In the absence of concerning findings, however, rupture of membranes is inappropriate and the pregnancy should be continued and monitored as in the explanation for A.

E. The patient should be instructed to follow fetal kick counts if she is discharged home after at least 4 hours of monitoring. However, this is not the most appropriate initial step in management.

6. | **B.** Pregnant women are volume expanded and often manifest signs of shock after greater loss of volume as compared to nonpregnant women. Any trauma patient presenting with seizures should be treated with magnesium sulfate and assessed rapidly for preeclampsia. Women with eclampsia, especially if they are driving, may sustain significant trauma.

A. US of the placenta identifies only 25% of abruptions, which must be quite large to be seen. Thus a normal US cannot be too reassuring. Abruptions are commonly identified retrospectively, after delivery of the placenta. Often, clinical decisions are guided by a suspicion for abruption based on symptoms and signs such as decreased fetal movement, nonreassuring fetal testing, and uterine contractions.

C. While a small subset of patients who suffer loss of consciousness (LOC) may need emergent cesarean delivery to enhance resuscitation, the best resuscitation for the fetus typically is to resuscitate the mother. Thus LOC alone is not an indication for emergent delivery.

D. The large gravid uterus impedes effective administration of CPR. Thus, if a pregnant patient in the third trimester requires CPR, generally an emergent cesarean delivery is required to improve the results of CPR.

E. The uterus and amniotic fluid protect the fetus during most blunt abdominal traumas. Thus injury to the fetus is rare.

7. **C.** One should have a low threshold to rule out rupture of membranes in any patient complaining of increased vaginal discharge. If missed, this condition may lead to significantly increased rates of infection and preterm delivery, in addition to potential loss of treatment options such as antibiotics and, if indicated, steroids for fetal lung maturity. The description of fluid "running down her legs" in this particular patient makes rupture of membranes the most likely etiology. A sterile speculum exam should be performed to examine the vagina for a "pool" of amnionic fluid, check the fluid's pH with nitrazine paper, and collect a small amount of fluid on a slide that should exhibit a ferning pattern when dried. If this patient does have rupture of membranes, the management would be immediate induction of labor to reduce the probability of maternal and neonatal infection.

A. Chlamydia should be screened for in a patient with the complaint of vaginal discharge. This is not the best answer to this question for two reasons: (1) The patient's complaint of watery discharge is less consistent with chlamydial infection and more consistent with rupture of membranes, bacterial vaginosis, trichomoniasis, or physiologic discharge. Generally, a chlamydial infection will lead to a more purulent discharge. (2) If this patient did rule out for rupture of membranes, a chlamydia DNA test has far higher sensitivity than a culture.

B. While the urine chlamydia test is a DNA test, it can be done after determining whether the patient has ruptured membranes, which is the more likely diagnosis.

D. Herpes infection generally presents with pain, burning or itching, and blistering lesions. It is not typically associated with increased vaginal discharge. If the patient has a history of herpes, one should have a low threshold for evaluation and culture, but this patient's symptoms do not suggest herpes.

E. In patients in whom the diagnosis of rupture of membranes is questionable, but the patient gives a very good history (as this patient does), it is reasonable to perform an US to look for amniotic fluid volume. In this patient, this step would be secondary to the primary diagnostic techniques for amnionic fluid leakage (i.e., sterile speculum exam).

8. **E.** The patient's symptoms and exam are consistent with an infected Bartholin's cyst, also called a Bartholin's abscess. The Bartholin's glands are found in the vulva, on both sides of the vaginal fourchette. They normally secrete mucin, which drains into the vagina. Obstruction of the duct leads to formation of a cyst. Infection of the cyst, or abscess formation, may occur rapidly. The infection tends to be polymicrobial, involving mixed bacterial organisms and sometimes *Neisseria gonorrhea*. A Bartholin's abscess must be drained. Drainage is accomplished with local anesthesia, a small incision, and drainage of the infected material. The abscess must be allowed to continue to drain. A Word catheter, with a balloon tip, may be placed to maintain patency of the abscess cavity.

A. A Bartholin's abscess is extremely uncomfortable, and the pain is immediately reduced significantly with drainage. Management with antibiotics alone is inappropriate. If the abscess is unrelated to *Neisseria gonorrhea*, the patient may not need antibiotics at all.

B. Hospitalization and treatment with IV antibiotics is unnecessary. Incision and drainage are most important, and likely curative.

C. A screen for STDs may be performed, but incision and drainage are the most important order of management. Bartholin's abscess was initially thought to be highly associated with *Neisseria gonorrhea*, but further data suggest that the association is not so strong.

D. Warm compresses will not help if the duct is blocked. In the days and weeks after the cyst has been incised, they may help to facilitate further drainage.

9. | **B.** Any woman of reproductive age with abnormal bleeding or spotting should be evaluated for pregnancy. Spotting can occur with implantation or—more concerning—can be a sign of ectopic pregnancy. If the patient is pregnant, she should be evaluated further with a pelvic US to confirm that the pregnancy is intrauterine and not ectopic.

A. Postcoital spotting can be a sign of cervical cancer, although cervical polyps or infections are more common. Patients should have Pap smears performed if they have not had one within the past year.

C. Cervical cultures should also be sent, after the urine pregnancy test.

D. Pelvic US is not indicated, unless the patient is pregnant.

E. A urinary tract infection may cause pink spotting, although this is rare.

10. | **A.** Midcycle spotting may be hormonal in origin, or may be caused by a lesion such as endometrial cancer, cervical or uterine polyps, or fibroids. Uterine cancer is often detected early because 90% of patients present with abnormal bleeding and can, therefore, be treated successfully. Women older than age 35 with unexplained, irregular bleeding should be evaluated by endometrial biopsy, with endocervical curettage.

B. While some patients with endometrial cancer will have abnormal Pap smears, most will have normal Pap smears. Regardless, the patient should be up-to-date on her Pap smears to ensure that she does not have cervical cancer.

C. Cervicitis and STDs can cause abnormal cervical bleeding. However, the patient must first be evaluated for endometrial cancer.

D. Pelvic US may add data on the thickness and contour of the endometrial stripe, suggesting a polyp or, especially among postmenopausal women, abnormal thickening. However, US is never diagnostic. In this case, tissue is important for diagnosis.

E. Hysteroscopy, looking for polyps, fibroids, or locations for directed biopsies, should be considered if the endometrial biopsy is normal.

11. | **C.** Uterine fibroids may distort the uterine cavity, impairing implantation or causing infertility. This patient has achieved pregnancy twice. Fibroids may be associated with spontaneous abortion, preterm labor, and infertility. The patient is 39 years old and her fertility will likely decline rapidly. Given her history, myomectomy is a reasonable option.

A. Consideration of adoption is a personal issue and one that is often discussed with patients undergoing infertility treatments. While adoption should be considered, myomectomy is a reasonable option that should be offered to the patient.

B. A gestational carrier is a woman who carries a pregnancy for another couple (a "surrogate mother"). The couple's own sperm and egg often create the pregnancy. This option is relevant to a woman who cannot carry a pregnancy, often because of anatomic problems such as cervical incompetence. Such an approach is controversial and often expensive. This patient's history does not suggest the need for a gestational carrier.

D. ICSI is reserved for situations in which the sperm is qualitatively or quantitatively unlikely to enter the egg on its own. This couple has a normal semen analysis and, more importantly, has achieved two pregnancies without ICSI. Thus they do not need this technology.

E. The patient has already been able to conceive, so IVF is unnecessary.

12. **B.** LSC is the result of an irritant causing pruritis and subsequent mechanical irritation (scratching) that leads to epidermal hyperplasia. On exam, the area appears diffusely red with hyperplastic or hyperpigmented plaques. Treatment includes topical steroids and antipruritics.

A. Eczema does not commonly occur on the vulva; common locations include the antecubital fossa and hands.

C. Lichen sclerosis is also characterized by vulvar pruritis and diffusely involves the vulva. In contrast to LSC, lesions are thin and whitish, commonly termed "onion skin" lesions. Furthermore, lichen sclerosis tends to occur in postmenopausal women, and occasionally in premenarchal girls, but rarely in women in their twenties. Treatment is topical steroids. This disorder poses no increased risk for vulvar carcinoma.

D, E. Melanoma, squamous cell carcinoma, and basal cell carcinoma are the three most common vulvar cancers, but are certainly much less common than LSC, particularly in this age group.

13. **B.** The incubation period for syphilis is 14 to 21 days. This patient has an early infection of syphilis with painless ulcerations on her labia. An ulcer or *chancre* may occur on any mucosal surface, including the vulva, vagina, penis, cervix, anus, nipples, and lips.

A. The treatment for early (less than 1 year) syphilis is a single intramuscular injection of benzathine penicillin. If syphilis has gone undetected for more than a year, three doses should be administered. Treatment for neurosyphilis includes aqueous crystalline penicillin G, 2–4 million units IV every 4 hours for nearly 2 weeks, followed by three weekly doses of benzathine penicillin.

C. Syphilis is caused by the spirochete *Treponema pallidum*.

D, E. Early syphilis can progress to secondary syphilis 1 to 3 months after initial infection as the chancres disappear and a characteristic maculopapular rash appears on the palms of the hands and soles of the feet. Syphilis, which is known as the "great imitator," may have a multitude of manifestations, including hepatitis, meningitis, and nephritis. If left untreated, the disease enters a latent phase, which is highly variable and may last for several years. The disease culminates in tertiary syphilis, which is characterized by skin gummas (granulomas), infection of the aorta (aortitis), and neurosyphilis with meningovascular disease; tabes dorsalis, and paresis. Notched teeth and saber shins are characteristics of neonatal syphilis rather than tertiary syphilis.

14. **A.** In this patient with very uncertain dates, obtaining evidence of fetal lung maturity is essential before actively initiating delivery. Because of the increased risks of traumatic birth due to macrosomia, and higher rates of intrauterine fetal demise, patients with gestational diabetes treated with insulin are regularly induced at 39 to 40 weeks. If dating is certain, assessment of fetal lung maturity is not necessary so close to term. Importantly, organ development, including lung maturity, in fetuses of diabetic mothers is actually delayed. Biochemical evidence of fetal lung maturity (e.g., amniotic fluid lecithin:sphingomyelin ratio) is needed, as the risk of respiratory distress syndrome may outweigh the risk of continued gestation.

B, C. An OGTT could formally establish a diagnosis of diabetes, which is hardly in question given the patient's extremely elevated fasting blood sugar. The HbA_{1c} level would allow assessment of blood glucose control over the last 1 to 2 months, and is almost certain to be elevated in this patient with untreated disease. Both measurements provide valuable information for the management of this patient, but neither will substantially alter obstetrical decisions made at this point. Blood sugars can be controlled with insulin, and the fetus should be delivered if fetal lung maturity is documented. Of note, although this patient does not give a history of overt diabetes, today's fasting glucose is highly suggestive of pregestational disease; the American Diabetes Association considers a fasting glucose level higher than 126 to be diagnostic of overt diabetes.

D. This patient's fetus is markedly macrosomic (more than 4500 g). Cervical exam would be critical if induction of labor for vaginal delivery was planned, but an estimated fetal weight exceeding 4500 g is an indication for cesarean delivery to avoid the incidence of shoulder dystocia and its sequelae.

E. Quantitative β-hCG would not be useful in managing this patient (although it should be noted for screening purposes that β-hCG is decreased in pregnancies complicated by diabetes).

15. **A.** Without significant proteinuria, this patient does not have evidence of preeclampsia. Thus, if no other etiology for her hypertension is identified, discharge home with oral hypertensives may be appropriate. Labetolol and Aldomet are generally considered first-line therapy in this situation. Aldomet (methyldopa) enjoys the benefit of the most clinical experience and is thought to be very safe, but is not a very effective antihypertensive. Labetolol is the beta blocker of choice in pregnancy, is more effective than Aldomet, and is also considered safe (there is some suggestion of intrauterine growth restriction with atenolol). Another agent that is increasingly used but is not an answer choice here is nifedipine, a calcium-channel blocker.

B, D. ACE inhibitors are contraindicated in pregnancy because of evidence for fetal renal toxicity when given in the second and third trimesters. Similarly, angiotensin receptor blockers are contraindicated in pregnancy.

C. Magnesium sulfate is used in preeclampsia for seizure prophylaxis; it does *not* treat hypertension.

E. Diuretics are generally avoided in pregnancy due to concerns about intravascular volume depletion. They are not absolutely contraindicated, but better options for control of hypertension exist.

16. **E.** Gestational hypertension is often a retrospective diagnosis, in which hypertension in pregnancy is not preceded by pregestational (chronic) hypertension and does not result in significant proteinuria (and thus is not a form of preeclampsia). As long as BPs normalize by 12 weeks postpartum, the patient can be reassured that she does not have chronic hypertension.

A, B. The diagnosis of preeclampsia requires proteinuria (300 mg on 24-hour collection) or repeated spot urine protein (more than 30 mg/dL, equivalent to 1+). Although urine protein can fluctuate, this patient was never observed to have significant proteinuria.

C, D. Chronic hypertension is defined as hypertension preceding pregnancy, or hypertension measured at less than 20 weeks GA. Chronic hypertension puts patients at increased risk for preeclampsia. This patient has evidence of neither chronic hypertension nor preeclampsia.

17. **A.** Classification of ovarian neoplasms is based on the cell of origin: surface epithelial, germ, or sex-cord stromal cells. Epithelial cell tumors are the most common (90% of malignant ovarian tumors and 65% to 70% of all ovarian tumors). Major categories of epithelial tumors include serous and mucinous tumors, endometrioid clear cell, undifferentiated carcinoma, and Brenner tumor.

B. While epithelial cell tumors can affect women age 20 and older, they are most frequently observed among women in their late fifties.

C, D. Germ cell tumors include teratomas, dysgerminomas, endodermal sinus tumors, and choriocarcinoma. They generally affect girls and women of 0 to 25 years of age. Like all tumors, however, they may be seen at any age.

E. The major types of sex-cord stromal tumors include granulosa-theca and Sertoli-Leydig cell tumors as well as gonadoblastomas.

18. **E.** Immature teratoma, a germ cell tumor, is derived from embryonic (fetal) tissue. In both types of teratomas, fat, hair, and bone can be seen. In Figure 18, hair can be seen consistent with a teratoma (most likely a mature teratoma).

A. Dysgerminomas arise from the undifferentiated germ cells.

B. Embryonal carcinoma includes the embryonic, yolk sac, and placental cell lines.

C. Endodermal sinus tumor arises from extraembryonic (yolk sac) tissue.

D. Choriocarcinoma arises from trophoblastic (placental) tissue.

19. | A. Dysgerminoma, a germ cell tumor of the ovary predominantly affecting girls and young women, is remarkable for its secretion of LDH as a tumor marker. Patients commonly present with a rapidly enlarging adnexal mass and abdominal pain.

B. Embryonal carcinomas may produce AFP, as well as hCG and CA-125.

C. Endodermal sinus tumors may produce AFP.

D. Choriocarcinoma is a germ cell tumor and also a form of gestational trophoblastic disease that secretes hCG.

E. Immature teratoma or immature dermoid cysts may produce CA-125.

20. | A. A "radical" mastectomy entails en bloc resection of the anterior chest, including resection of breast tissue, nipple-areolar complex, overlying skin, axillary lymph nodes, and pectoralis muscles; it is termed "modified" when pectoralis major is spared. The modified radical mastectomy is often the procedure chosen for node-positive disease, as it offers cosmetic advantages with equivalent disease-free and overall survival rates.

B. Total (simple) mastectomy includes resection of breast tissue, nipple-areolar complex, and overlying skin, but spares lymph nodes. It is often used for ductal carcinoma in situ (DCIS) or lobular carcinoma in situ (LCIS). When combined with radiation therapy, results are comparable to those achieved with radical procedures for these localized malignancies. Total mastectomy is not appropriate for node-positive disease.

C. Subcutaneous mastectomy includes resection of breast tissue only, sparing the nipple-areolar complex, skin, and lymph nodes. It is not indicated for treatment of breast cancer.

D. See the explanation for A.

E. Wide local excision entails breast-conserving removal of the tumor ("local") with tumor-free margins ("wide"). Appropriate candidates for this procedure are patients who have tumors smaller than 4 cm, no fixation to muscle or the chest wall, no involvement of the overlying skin, no multicentric lesions, and no fixed lymph nodes. This patient is not an appropriate candidate.

21. | B. Younger women with more aggressive tumors generally respond best to chemotherapy, especially if the tumor is hormone receptor negative (as in this patient). The standard adjuvant treatment for node-positive premenopausal women includes 6 months of CMF combination therapy, regardless of hormone-receptor status.

A. Hormonal therapy is less effective in hormone-receptor–negative tumors, but some response is seen. Hormonal therapy may, in fact, be the preferred choice for an older patient prioritizing quality of life in the short term, as these agents are better tolerated than chemotherapeutic agents and are often better for palliative therapy.

C. Strontium is sometimes used as a bone-targeting isotope for multifocal bone metastases. This patient shows no evidence of bone metastases.

D. Herceptin is a monoclonal antibody directed against the c-erbB-2 signal transduction protein. This patient does not overexpress this protein and is unlikely to benefit from this therapy.

E. See the explanation for B.

22.   **D.** Medullary carcinoma is more frequent in younger patients and, despite being rather aggressive, carries a relatively favorable prognosis. Tubular carcinoma and mucinous (colloid) carcinoma are other, less common subtypes that carry better prognoses than intraductal carcinoma.

A, B. Tumors that are positive for hormone receptors carry more favorable prognoses.

C. Aneuploid tumors with a high S-phase fraction tend to be more aggressive and carry poorer prognoses than diploid tumors with a low S-phase fraction. It should be noted that tumor stage is more predictive than histology in determining prognosis.

E. Premenopausal women tend to have more aggressive disease and higher associated mortality.

23.   **D.** The TNM system stages breast malignancies by the size of the primary tumor (T), regional nodal involvement (N), and distant metastases (M). This patient has a tumor larger than 2 cm but smaller than 5 cm (T2), metastases to the axillary lymph nodes that are fixed (N2), and no evidence of distant metastasis (M0). This corresponds to stage grouping IIIa.

A, B, C, E. See the explanation for D and Table 23.

■ TABLE 23	TNM Classification of Breast Cancer
T: Primary Tumor	
T_x	Primary tumor unassessable
T_0	No evidence of primary tumor
T_{is}	Carcinoma in situ
T_1	< 2 cm
T_2	> 2 cm, < 5 cm
T_3	> 5 cm
T_4	Any tumor extending to the chest wall or skin
N: Regional Lymph Nodes	
N_x	Regional lymph nodes cannot be assessed
N_0	No regional lymph node metastases
N_1	Metastasis to mobile ipsilateral axillary node
N_2	Metastasis to ipsilateral axillary node, fixed
N_3	Metastasis to ipsilateral internal mammary node
M: Distant Metastases	
M_x	Presence of distant metastasis cannot be assessed
M_0	No evidence of distant metastasis
M_1	Distant metastasis

24. | E. This young woman has PID. She should be admitted to the hospital and receive intravenous antibiotics as she is unable to tolerate oral medications and has failed outpatient management. She has many risk factors for PID, including some of the following: age (15- to 19-year-old age group), early onset of sexual activity, and multiple partners. Other risk factors may include partner infection with gonorrhea or chlamydia, personal history of recurrent STDs, personal history of PID, douching, and even cigarette smoking, all of which have been shown to increase the risk of contracting PID. Barrier contraception appears to be protective against PID.

A. If this patient does not improve within 24 to 48 hours with IV antibiotics, a pelvic US may be obtained to diagnose tubo-ovarian abscess(es), but is unnecessary at this point.

B. A urine pregnancy test routinely can detect an elevated serum β-hCG of 20 or more, so obtaining a serum β-hCG is not necessary in this case. In the future, secondary to this episode of PID, the patient is at risk for ectopic pregnancy (as well as infertility and pelvic pain).

C. This patient is not a candidate for outpatient management of her infection. She has failed an outpatient regimen due to noncompliance and is unable to tolerate oral medications. Other contraindications to outpatient management would include pregnancy, an immunocompromised state, a pelvic abscess, or a patient with a surgical abdomen.

D. Laparoscopy has been used as the "gold standard" to make the diagnosis of PID in small clinical studies. However, it is rarely used in this way because of the risks of surgery. Laparoscopy would be reasonable in a patient with tubo-ovarian abscess that is resistant to intravenous antibiotics or that has ruptured.

25. | C. The patient has post-IUD insertion endometritis or an infection of the endometrium. When the infection spreads into the myometrium, it is called endomyometritis. There is considerable overlap with the diagnosis of PID—only the clinical situation differentiates them. Risk factors include instrumentation of some type such as IUD insertion, D&C or D&E, normal spontaneous vaginal delivery, or cesarean section. In addition to pain and tenderness, affected patients often have a fever and leukocytosis. The best course of management is removal of the IUD and antibiotics. The antibiotics of choice are identical to those used to treat PID.

A. This patient does not have any contraindications for outpatient management of endometritis, and it is safe to treat her with an outpatient regimen. The CDC currently recommends the following: oral ofloxacin (400 mg PO BID) or levofloxacin (500 mg PO QD) with or without metronidazole (500 mg PO BID); another regimen involves ceftriaxone (250 mg IM once) or cefoxitin (2 g IM once) plus probenecid (1 g PO once) followed by doxycycline (100 mg PO BID) with or without metronidazole (500 mg PO BID). This treatment should last 14 days.

B. Oral antibiotics are appropriate only after the foreign body is removed.

D. Repeat cultures are unlikely to be positive and would not change the management. Additionally, the treatment you provide would eradicate any gonorrhea and chlamydia present. This infection likely resulted from contamination of the

IUD with bacteria from the vagina or cervix. NSAIDs would be helpful for pain management.

E. The patient is not likely to be pregnant. A pregnancy test is usually obtained at insertion time. Additionally, she reports no intercourse in more than 4 weeks. It is important to remember that if she does get pregnant, she is at increased risk for an ectopic pregnancy.

26. | **B.** Emergency contraception formulations have a relative failure rate of approximately 25%. Therefore, these pills decrease a woman's absolute pregnancy risk from 8% to 2%. Progestin-only pills fare slightly better, having a relative failure rate of 11%. The most common side effect of either regimen is nausea, although the side-effect rate is much higher with preparations including estrogen.

A. Any of the emergency contraception types can be used up to 72 hours after the time of unprotected sexual intercourse.

C. Emergency contraception can be obtained from a variety of sources, including primary care doctors, pharmacists, local community clinics, and Internet Web sites.

D. Numerous studies have shown that OCPs taken inadvertently during pregnancy pose no threat to the developing embryo. This is generally believed to be true regarding emergency contraception as well.

E. Prior use of an IUD has no bearing on the effectiveness of emergency contraception.

27. | **C.** The patient has a tissue diagnosis and needs treatment for her disease. The appropriate treatment is a LEEP. This patient is not a candidate for cryotherapy (see the explanation for E).

A. A hysterectomy is too aggressive and not warranted given the pathology report.

B. A colposcopy is generally considered a diagnostic tool as opposed to a treatment for dysplasia and is not the standard of care after a tissue diagnosis of HSIL.

D. This patient does not need radiation therapy. Radiation therapy is the mainstay treatment for bulky advanced disease, not disease that is confined to the cervix.

E. This patient is not a candidate for cryotherapy because the transformation zone was not visualized in its entirety at the time of colposcopy; thus the patient needs a LEEP. A colposcopy is termed "satisfactory" only if the entire TZ is visualized. An "unsatisfactory" colposcopy is one of the three indications for a LEEP as opposed to cryotherapy; the other two are a positive ECC and a two-step discrepancy between the Pap smear and biopsy results.

28. | **C.** Fetal kidneys are examined on a routine obstetric US. Of note, renal pelvis dilation has been associated with aneuploidy and urinary obstruction. A Level I US usually includes location of pregnancy (i.e., intrauterine versus ectopic), location of placenta, amniotic fluid assessment, fetal lie, fetal biometric data for dating, and basic fetal anatomy. The anatomy scan routinely identifies cerebral landmarks such as the ventricles, thalamus, cerebellar hemispheres and posterior fossa, four-chamber view of the heart, stomach, spine, kidneys, bladder, and umbilical cord insertion.

A. Examining fetal extremities is not a part of the routine Level I US.

B. Despite the fact that many patients hope to find out fetal gender at the 18- to 22-week Level I US, it may be easily disclosed in only 80% to 90% of cases, and is not a component of the routine obstetric US.

D. While an image of the umbilical cord insertion into the fetal abdomen is important to rule out omphalocele, its insertion into the placenta is not a routine component of the obstetric US.

E. The fetal face is not a routine component of the Level I obstetric US.

29. **E.** D&E is most appropriate for this patient. It involves serial dilation of the cervix, followed by manual removal of fetal parts and placenta using specialized forceps and suction, as well as sharp curettage of the uterus. D&E is very effective for mid-trimester pregnancies up to 18 weeks GA, and can be done on an outpatient basis with less invasive anesthesia. While risks for adverse events including hemorrhage, perforation, and infection exist, this method has proven to be safest among the mid-trimester abortion methods such as vaginal prostaglandins or hypertonic saline instillation.

A. Suction curettage involves the use of a cannula attached to pump suction that is placed in the uterine cavity to suction out intrauterine contents. It usually requires a small amount of cervical dilation and is the most widely used method of induced abortion in the world. It has a very low risk of adverse events. However, sole use of this method is generally effective only in pregnancies up to approximately 12 weeks GA, after which time D&E is usually necessary.

B. Placement of prostaglandins such as prostaglandin E_2 in the vagina causes abortion via labor induction. The agent is administered every 3 to 4 hours until delivery has occurred. This procedure is appropriate for mid-trimester abortions, but is more time-consuming and associated with higher maternal morbidity than D&E.

C. Menstrual regulation involves the aspiration of endometrium within 14 days of a missed period or by 42 days after the beginning of the LMP. This safe and quick procedure can be done in the doctor's office, usually without anesthesia. It is a reliable and relatively inexpensive means of abortion. However, it must be done almost immediately after pregnancy is suspected to be effective, and is therefore not applicable to this patient.

D. Hysterectomy is not a method of pregnancy termination, particularly in this young patient who will likely desire preservation of fertility. Also, hysterectomy is generally not indicated in any patient unless other attempts at mid-trimester abortion have failed or the patient suffers from comorbid conditions, such as cervical stenosis, that would be satisfactorily addressed with hysterectomy.

30. **E.** The copper-T IUD is the most efficacious form of contraception for this patient. Given her need for long-term contraception, she would benefit most from a method that does not involve daily interventions. Of the two listed (Depo-Provera and the copper-T IUD), the IUD has not been associated with mood disturbances, likely because it is a physical device as opposed to a hormonal barrier. Depo-Provera, by contrast, utilizes hormonal agents and has been associated with depressive symptoms. This association is especially prominent among women with a history of postpartum depression, although any history of mood disorders warrants avoidance of Depo-Provera as a contraceptive method.

A. See the explanation for E.

B. Given her smoking history and age greater than 35 years, combination OCPs are contraindicated in this patient, as they significantly raise the risk of DVT, pulmonary embolism, and stroke. Daily regimens increase the chance of missed doses, and because this patient will presumably not want a quick reversal of contraception in the future, there is no need to keep that as an option. With proper use, however, combination OCPs offer the best protection overall, with a theoretical failure rate of 0.1%.

C. Progestin-only OCPs are even more restrictive than combination OCPs, needing to be taken within a very specific time window every day to work. Also, their failure rate is higher—0.5%.

D. The diaphragm is similarly a daily affair, and the failure rate is quite high at 6%.

31.
> **E.** Impaired hepatic function is considered an absolute contraindication to combination OCPs. Other absolute contraindications include thrombophlebitis, cerebral/coronary vascular disease, hyperlipidemia, undiagnosed vaginal bleeding, smoking if greater than 35 years old, pregnancy, known or suspected breast cancer, and hepatic neoplasm.

A. Vascular disease mediated by diabetes mellitus (DM) can be exacerbated by combination OCPs; in patients younger than 35, however, the risks of pregnancy outweigh the risks of this potential vascular pathology. Thus DM is only a relative contraindication in this case.

B. HTN is only a relative contraindication. If the patient is younger than 35 and her BP is well controlled, the benefits of contraception outweigh risks.

C. In the past, fibroids were considered a contraindication; however, modern combination OCPs have sufficiently low doses of estrogen to render fibroid growth unaffected.

D. Only a personal history of breast cancer is a contraindication. Family history is not considered to be a contraindication.

32.
> **A.** This patient presents with metastatic choriocarcinoma. Appropriate treatment for patients without "poor prognosis" risk factors is single-agent chemotherapy. Choriocarcinoma is a malignant, necrotizing tumor arising from trophoblastic tissue. It is often rapidly metastatic, spreading hematogenously to the lungs (most commonly) and also to the vagina, pelvis, brain, liver, and kidneys. Left untreated, this rapid metastasis can result in death within months. Fortunately, like other forms of gestational trophoblastic disease (GTD), choriocarcinoma is exquisitely sensitive to chemotherapy. Single-agent therapy is indicated for patients with nonmetastatic disease and patients with metastatic disease with no "poor prognosis" risk factors. Choriocarcinoma is one of the few malignancies where single-agent therapy remains the standard of care in modern medicine. It is important to note that only 50% of choriocarcinomas develop after a preceding molar pregnancy; 25% follow normal term pregnancy, and 25% follow ectopic pregnancy or abortion.

B. Multiple-agent chemotherapy is indicated for patients with metastatic choriocarcinoma and "poor prognosis" risk factors—namely, duration of disease greater than 4 months, serum β-hCG greater than 40,000, metastasis to the brain or liver, choriocarcinoma following term pregnancy, or unsuccessful single-agent chemotherapy. This patient does not have any of these risk factors.

C. Hysterectomy has a very limited role in choriocarcinoma, as the tumor is highly sensitive to chemotherapy and is often metastatic. Hysterectomy is an option only for patients who do not desire future fertility and who show no evidence of metastatic disease, but it results in a higher complication rate. This procedure is the treatment of choice for placental-site trophoblastic tumors, which are extremely rare tumors arising from the placental implantation site. Surgery is indicated for these patients because the tumor is poorly responsive to chemotherapy and rarely metastatic.

D, E. Because GTD is sensitive to chemotherapy and often metastatic, surgical intervention and radiation do not generally play a role in its treatment.

33. | **E.** Treatment of molar pregnancy consists of immediate evacuation of the uterus, followed by monitoring for persistent trophoblastic proliferation by serial β-hCG levels. This follow-up period should last at least one year, during which time reliable contraception is required to allow accurate measurement. The method of contraception is not critical, but OCPs offer the advantages of high efficacy and low incidence of irregular bleeding (which could be confused with persistent disease).

A. While it is true that the risk of GTD in future pregnancies is higher for this patient than for members of the general population (about 1% versus 0.1%), prompt diagnosis has reduced the mortality from molar pregnancies to near zero and morbidity to an acceptable level. The risk is not considered sufficiently high to discourage future pregnancy beyond the period required for monitoring of β-hCG levels.

B. Patients who are cured of molar pregnancy have no increase in the rate of spontaneous abortions, complications, or congenital malformations in future (nonmolar) pregnancies.

C, D. The risk of persistent and/or malignant trophoblastic disease is estimated at about 5% for a partial (incomplete) mole and 20% for a complete mole. OCPs do not reduce this risk (in fact, a weak association may exist between OCP use and persistent disease).

34. | **A.** Roughly 5% of all pregnancies are complicated by asymptomatic bacteriuria of more than 100,000 colonies on culture. The incidence of asymptomatic bacteriuria during pregnancy is similar to that for the nonpregnant population. During pregnancy, however, urinary stasis increases due to progesterone-induced relaxation of the ureters and bladder, and direct obstruction by the uterus. Consequently, pregnant women with untreated asymptomatic bacteriuria are more likely to develop UTIs, cystitis, and, most seriously, pyelonephritis. In 15% of pregnant patients with pyelonephritis, severe complications occur such as bacteremia, sepsis, and adult respiratory distress syndrome (ARDS). Because asymptomatic bacteriuria can progress to severe infection in the pregnant patient, it should be evaluated further—in this case, with a urine culture.

B. Symptoms of UTI during pregnancy may be somewhat nonspecific. Increased blood flow to the bladder and pressure from the uterus cause most pregnant women to experience frequency and sometimes urgency. Pregnant women may develop pyelonephritis without any preceding symptoms of UTI.

C. Vaginal flora and discharge may explain the urine dip results. Treating all patients presumptively with antibiotics will lead to increased microbial resistance, allergic reactions, and maternal side effects. Patients with a history of pyelonephritis, urologic surgery, or frequent UTIs may require suppressive therapy during pregnancy.

D. To ignore a urine dip suggestive of a UTI might result in progression of asymptomatic bacteriuria to pyelonephritis.

E. There is no indication for renal biopsy in this situation.

35. E. The patient has clear signs of chorioamnionitis, or infection of the chorion and amnion. Chorioamnionitis is the most common cause of neonatal sepsis, which poses a significant risk for neonatal death or cerebral palsy. Given the signs and the risks, and despite the early GA, the patient should be delivered. The patient should also be treated with intravenous fluids, Tylenol, and broad-spectrum antibiotics that include coverage for group B *Streptococcus*.

A. Cesarean section in this setting should be reserved for a persistently nonreassuring fetal heart tracing, malpresentation, or failed induction. A cesarean section in the setting of chorioamnionitis is associated with increased postpartum complications such as wound infection, abscess, and fistula formation.

B. The patient should receive antibiotics, but observation in the setting of diagnosed chorioamnionitis is inappropriate.

C. Amniocentesis for culture is sometimes performed when the diagnosis is unclear. In this case, the patient clearly has chorioamnionitis. Amniocentesis for culture would merely waste critical time.

D. The tampon dye test involves the placement of a tampon in the vagina with injection of indigo carmine into the amniotic cavity; the tampon is removed 1 hour later. Blue dye on the tampon confirms rupture of membranes. In this patient's case, the diagnosis of ruptured membranes has already been made by history, the ferning pattern caused by the high sodium concentration in the amniotic fluid, the nitrazine test, and the oligohydramnios, making the tampon dye test unnecessary.

36. B. The patient's symptoms are concerning for ruptured membranes, the most ominous of the possibilities suggested by the tests. Some patients leak fluid slowly after membrane rupture; as such, any patient complaining of vaginal wetness should be evaluated for membrane rupture. A sterile speculum must be used to reduce the risk of infection if the membranes have indeed ruptured. A pool of fluid may not be seen if the patient has a high leak or oligohydramnios. Fluid loss may be provoked by asking the patient to cough during the exam. Amniotic fluid contains a high concentration of sodium, which crystallizes on a slide when it dries, creating a fern-like pattern. Amniotic fluid is basic and should turn pH paper blue. If all tests are negative, and the suspicion for ruptured membranes is high, an US should be performed to check the amniotic fluid index. A tampon dye test may be performed if the suspicion for rupture is high but the above-mentioned tests are negative.

A. Observation at home when rupture of membranes is suggested by history is inappropriate initial evaluation and inappropriate management if rupture is confirmed and the fetus is viable.

C. In addition to evaluation for ruptured membranes, the patient should be checked with a wet prep to rule out bacterial vaginosis or a candidal infection. Either could explain her symptoms.

D. A Group B *Streptococcus* culture is appropriate for any patient at risk for preterm delivery. In this case, however, one must first assess membrane status.

E. US may be performed to assess fluid as part of the evaluation for ruptured membranes. First, however, one must perform a sterile speculum exam to assess for leakage of fluid.

37.
> **E.** This patient has been exposed to VZV, or chickenpox, and is at risk because she may not have had the disease before. Chickenpox during pregnancy can be severe, carrying as high as a 25% risk of maternal mortality should varicella pneumonia develop. If the patient contracts varicella infection 5 days before or after delivery, the neonate is at risk for life-threatening neonatal varicella infection. This patient is within 72 hours of the time of exposure, so she may benefit from VZIG if she has never had varicella. Fortunately, 70% to 90% of patients who think they have never had chickenpox show detectable antibodies, and thus do not need VZIG. Rapid VZV screening for prior exposure is available. The patient should go to an area of the ED designated for patients with exposures to potentially infectious diseases and have a VZV titer drawn. If the titer is negative, she should return later in the day for VZIG. You should call the ED and alert them that she is coming.

A. The patient must be advised to avoid the clinic, where she could potentially infect other pregnant women.

B. While the patient qualifies for VZIG because she is within the 72-hour window, she may not need passive immunity if she has previously had the disease. A rapid VZV titer should be drawn prior to VZIG administration.

C. Oral acyclovir, when administered within 24 hours of the appearance of the rash, may reduce the duration of new lesion formation and the total number of lesions. Oral acyclovir is safe in pregnancy and may provide symptomatic relief. It does not reduce the risk of vertical transmission. This patient is not clearly infected with varicella and prescription of acyclovir is premature.

D. VZIG should be given to infants born to women who develop a varicella infection between 5 days prior to and 2 days after delivery. If this patient develops varicella infection and delivers within 5 days, the pediatrician needs to be alerted and the infant prophylaxed.

38.
> **C.** The RPR and the VDRL are both nonspecific antibody screening tests for *T. pallidum*, or syphilis. Diagnosis is confirmed with either the more specific microhemagglutination assay for antibodies to *T. pallidum* (MHA-TP) or the fluorescent treponemal antibody-absorption (FTA-ABS) technique. Nonspecific screening tests such as the RPR or the VDRL yield many false-positives and must be followed with confirmatory testing before action is taken. In this case, sending an MHA-TP is appropriate. Because congenital syphilis can be quite severe and treatment for syphilis is available, this infection is screened for universally in pregnancy.

A, B. Patients with rheumatologic disease may falsely screen positive for syphilis and are sometimes identified this way. This patient's intermittent arthritis and fatigue are somewhat nonspecific, and she may merit further evaluation for rheumatologic disease. However, evaluation for syphilis is the most appropriate next step.

D. Confirmatory testing is needed prior to treatment, with the possible exception of a case involving a highly noncompliant patient at high risk for syphilis (e.g., with a known positive partner).

E. Rather than repeat a nonspecific test, one should send the more specific confirmatory test. Repeating the RPR merely wastes time. A negative result would not erase the fact that the first test was positive and would simply raise concerns for a false-negative or a lab error.

39. | **B.** Domestic violence increases during pregnancy, and occurs in 4% to 8% of pregnancies. The perpetrator is usually a current or prior intimate partner. A controlling partner and multiple somatic complaints may be present. Domestic violence often goes unrecognized, and universal screening must be undertaken. This patient's frequent, nonspecific complaints suggest that she is reaching out for help. She needs to be asked about domestic violence in a supportive manner. Studies have shown that most women support and appreciate universal inquiry about domestic violence. Examples of screening questions include the following:
    - Has anyone close to you ever threatened to hurt you?
    - Have you ever been afraid of your partner?
    - Do you feel safe at home?
    - Has anyone ever hit, kicked, choked, or hurt you physically?
    - Has anyone, including your partner, ever forced you to have sex?

A. The biophysical profile is typically used to follow up a nonreactive NST.

C. The patient should be asked about her weight gain in a supportive manner. The Institute of Medicine recommends that normal-weight women gain between 25 and 35 lb during pregnancy. Maternal weight gain often occurs most rapidly during the third trimester.

D, E. There is no indication for US or weekly nonstress tests at this point.

40. | **D.** In addition to breast enlargement, the patient has a secondary mound caused by projection of the areola and papilla. This is characteristic of Tanner stage 4 (see Figure 40a). In addition, her pubic hair appears mid-escutcheon, characteristic of Tanner stage 4. The patient's exam suggests the presence of circulating estrogens, as well as normal anatomy, both of which are important in the evaluation of primary amenorrhea.

A, B, C, E. Preadolescent breasts, with elevation of the papilla only, characterize Tanner stage 1. Pubic hair is absent. Breast buds characterize Tanner stage 2. The breast and papilla are elevated, and the areola is engorged. Presexual axillary and pubic hair may be present. Tanner stage 3 is characterized by further development of breast size, without separation in contour from the breast and the areola. Axillary and sexual pubic hair may be present. Tanner stage 5 is the mature stage. The breasts have an adult contour, with recession of the areola. Axillary hair and a female escutcheon are present. Figure 40b depicts Tanner stages 1, 2, 3, 5.

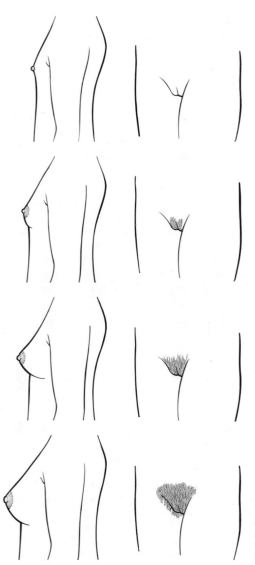

Figure 40b • Reproduced with permission from Callahan T. Blueprints Obstetrics & Gynecology. 3rd ed. Blackwell, 2004: Figs. 20-2 and 20-3, p. 181.

41.   **D.** The most common cause of secondary amenorrhea is pregnancy. This patient reports that she's never been sexually active, and her urine pregnancy test is negative. The patient is extremely thin, and she must be evaluated for anorexia nervosa. Weight loss, anorexia nervosa, stress, and exercise can all cause hypothalamic dysfunction and disruption in the pulsatile secretion of GnRH, resulting in hypogonadotropic hypogonadism. Most adolescents experience some degree of hypothalamic amenorrhea during the first few years after menarche.

A. Cervical stenosis can lead to secondary amenorrhea and is usually caused by scarring of the cervical os as a result of obstetric trauma or surgery; this patient has had neither.

B. Asherman's syndrome is the presence of intrauterine synechiae or adhesions and is usually caused by infection or surgery. D&C, cesarean section, myomectomy, and endometritis, which are not part of this patient's history, may lead to Asherman's syndrome.

C. POF is defined by menopause that occurs before age 40. Chromosomal analysis is sent before the age of 35 to rule out a genetic basis for POF. It may result from radiation, chemotherapy, infection, or ovarian surgery, but is most often idiopathic. While it is a possible diagnosis in this case, the patient has no other symptoms of menopause, and POF is not the most likely diagnosis.

E. PCOS, originally described as Stein-Leventhal syndrome, represents a spectrum of disease characterized by oligomenorrhea and some degree of chemical or clinical androgenization. While it is a possible diagnosis in this case, the patient has no evidence of androgenization, and it is not the most likely diagnosis.

42. **A.** Metronidazole (Flagyl), dosed orally at 2 g once, is often sufficient treatment for *Trichomonas vaginalis*, the infection from which this patient suffers. The presence of actively moving, flagellated organisms seen on wet prep is diagnostic of *Trichomonas* infection.

B. Partners must always be treated or they will continue to pass the infection back and forth to each other.

C. Alternative treatment for *Trichomonas* infection includes azithromycin (Zithromax) at 1 g orally given once.

D. Any patient diagnosed with an STD is at risk for all STDs and needs full screening.

E. Diagnosis of *Trichomonas vaginalis* infection can be made based on wet prep alone. A culture is unnecessary when the wet prep is positive, and may result in delayed treatment or lost treatment opportunity.

43. **B.** This patient's presentation strongly suggests cervicitis, and not PID, likely caused by infection with *Neisseria gonorrhoeae* (GC) or *Chlamydia trachomatis*. GC can be treated by a single dose of ceftriaxone; CT can be treated with either a single dose of azithromycin (1 g) or a 7-day course of doxycycline. Some small studies support a 2-g dose to treat GC as well as CT. If left untreated, cervicitis may progress to PID. The three major criteria used to diagnose PID are abdominal pain, adnexal pain, and cervical motion tenderness; this patient has only cervical motion tenderness. Hospitalization and treatment with IV antibiotics would constitute overtreatment and are not indicated in the setting of uncomplicated cervicitis. Cervical cultures should be performed prior to presumptive treatment. The patient's partner also needs treatment. In addition, this patient should be counseled to use condoms because of their relative protection against STDs, and she should be offered full STD screening, including an HIV test. Among sexually active women, 20- to 24-year-olds have the highest prevalence of gonococcal and chlamydial infections.

A. While ceftriaxone covers GC, it does not cover CT adequately, and these infections can often occur together.

C. Doxycycline does not adequately cover GC.

D. As noted in the explanation for B, a 2-g regimen has some coverage for GC, but a 1-g dose is not the standard recommended regimen to cover GC.

E. IV cefoxitin and doxycycline are appropriate for inpatient treatment of PID.

44. **D.** Uterine fibroids are the sole cause of infertility in 2% to 10% of cases. Fibroid-related infertility may be due to distortion of the endocervical canal, endometrial cavity, or fallopian tubes, which interferes with conception or implantation and may cause spontaneous abortion.

A. An estimated 20% to 30% of American women develop fibroids by age 40, and 50% to 65% have no clinical symptoms. The most common symptom is abnormal vaginal bleeding, as seen in this patient. Pressure-related symptoms are relatively common as well. Symptoms generally depend on the location of the fibroids. In this patient, the posterior location of her fairly large fibroid has also caused dyspareunia and constipation.

B. Studies suggest that the degeneration of a fibroid to a leiomyosarcoma occurs rarely, on the order of 1 in 1000 cases. Rapidly enlarging fibroids in women who are postmenopausal or who have uncertain diagnoses are causes for concern. The decision to perform myomectomy, however, is often not based on a concern for malignant potential.

C. Estrogen stimulates fibroid growth, causing some fibroids to increase significantly during pregnancy and to regress after menopause. Fibroid growth during pregnancy may cause infarction and severe pain as a fibroid outgrows its blood supply. Fibroids may also cause intrauterine growth restriction (IUGR), uterine distortion causing fetal malpresentation, preterm labor, and dystocia, or blockage of the presenting part necessitating a cesarean section.

E. African American women have three to nine times the incidence of uterine fibroids as compared to Hispanic, Asian, and Caucasian women.

45. **B.** CIN II, or moderate dysplasia, also described as high-grade squamous intraepithelial lesion (HSIL), may progress to cervical cancer if left untreated. Destruction or excision of the lesion is needed. The endocervical curettage was performed to assess the endocervical canal, which cannot be viewed during colposcopy. This patient has no abnormal tissue identified by endocervical curettage. Her lesions are small, non-invasive, and confined to the exocervix, making her a candidate for cryotherapy or laser therapy. She will still require follow-up. See Table 45.

A. HPV infection is the primary cause of cervical cancer and premalignant lesions. Virus serotypes 16, 18, and 31 are especially closely correlated with cervical cancer. HPV serotype testing is currently used at some institutions to direct management of Pap smears read out as atypical squamous cells of undetermined significance

TABLE 45	Management of Abnormal Pap Smears
Abnormality		**Treatment**
ASC-US		HPV serotype testing • If (+) for high-risk HPV: colposcopy • If (−) for high-risk HPV: repeat Pap smear in 1 year
ASC-H		Colposcopy
LSIL	CIN I (mild dysplasia)	Colposcopy • If confirmed LSIL on colposcopic biopsy: colposcopy every 4 to 6 months • If persistent LSIL (more than 1 to 2 years) on colposcopy: ° Confined to exocervix: cryotherapy, laser therapy, or LEEP ° Involving endocervical canal: cervical conization via LEEP or CKC
HSIL	CIN II (moderate dysplasia)	Colposcopy • If confirmed HSIL on colposcopic biopsy:
	CIN III (severe dysplasia)	° Confined to exocervix: cryotherapy, laser therapy, or LEEP ° Involving endocervical canal: cervical conization via LEEP or CKC

ASC-US: Atypical squamous cells of undetermined significance.
HPV: Human papillomavirus.
ASC-H: Atypical squamous cells, cannot exclude high-grade squamous intraepithelial lesion.
LSIL: Low-grade squamous intraepithelial lesion.
CIN: Cervical intraepithelial neoplasia.
LEEP: Loop electrosurgical excision procedure (removing a cone-shaped piece of cervix with a cauterized wire loop).
CKC: Cold knife cone biopsy (removal of a wedge-shaped portion of the cervical stroma and endocervical canal).
HSIL: High-grade squamous intraepithelial lesion.

(ASC-US). However, because CIN II already represents precancerous changes (i.e., HSIL), further testing for HPV serotype would not alter the patient's management.

C, D. LEEP and CKC are generally performed when CIN II or III involves the endocervix, or when there is a discrepancy between the Pap smear and colposcopy.

E. Patients with ASC-US and CIN I may be followed with colposcopy every 3 to 4 months. If left untreated, approximately 30% of CIN I lesions will resolve. It takes about 7 years for CIN I lesions to progress to cervical cancer.

46.

B. A complex ovarian mass in a postmenopausal woman is highly suspicious for cancer and requires a diagnostic and staging laparotomy. The patient's signs and symptoms—in particular, a complex mass in the setting of ascites—are particularly concerning for ovarian cancer. The US image shows a large ovarian mass that is both cystic and solid. The worrisome finding on the image suggestive of malignancy is the appearance of the internal excrescences. Exploratory laparotomy is performed for diagnosis and, if cancer is found, for staging and debulking of the tumor.

A. The postmenopausal ovary does not cycle. A complex ovarian cyst in a post-menopausal woman is highly suspicious for carcinoma and is not expected to re-solve. A delay in diagnosis is potentially harmful.

C. Diuretic treatment of ascites has little efficacy, as fluid reaccumulates. When fluid returns to the third space, the patient may become intravascularly depleted and dehydrated. Thus diuretic treatment of ascites can be harmful.

D. A second opinion is reserved for cases in which management is unclear or con-troversial, which is not applicable here. A patient may always seek a second opinion herself, a move that should be supported.

E. If ovarian carcinoma is found, the patient will undergo a surgical debulking of her tumor followed by chemotherapy. Until an accurate tissue diagnosis is made, chemotherapy should not be given. Debulking the tumor is also thought to increase the percentage of tumor in the S phase, making the tumor relatively more responsive to chemotherapy than the patient's normal tissue.

47. | **C.** The image shown in the US depicts the fetal head in a case of a neural tube de-fect known as spina bifida. The two anomalies seen in the image are the "lemon" sign, which is exhibited by the concavities of the frontal bones, and the "banana" sign, evidenced by the abnormal shape of the cerebellum. While the defect in spina bifida is usually one of the lower spinal cord, it can be difficult to diag-nose on US directly. Rather, the findings in the fetal brain tend to make the US diagnosis. Spina bifida was the first fetal anomaly to be screened for with mater-nal serum screening. Mothers with fetuses who have neural tube defects have an elevated MSAFP, but the other analytes (estriol and hCG) should be normal.

A. Decreased MSAFP, decreased estriol, and an elevated hCG are seen in fetuses with Down syndrome. US findings in cases of Down syndrome include a short humerus and femur, the "double bubble" sign of duodenal atresia, endocardial cush-ion defects, nuchal thickening, and soft findings of echogenic intracardiac focus and pyelectasis. Notably, nearly 50% of Down syndrome fetuses will have a normal US.

B. Fetuses with trisomy 18 may have a decrease in all three analytes in the XAFP.

D, E. These two patterns of XAFP analytes are not associated with any particular syndrome.

48. | **E.** The patient has a small, functional cyst, which will most likely resolve spon-taneously. Cysts that are larger than 5 cm pose a significantly increased risk of ovarian torsion, of which this patient has no symptoms.

A. Combination OCPs reduce the likelihood of formation of new cysts through suppression of ovulation, but will not cause the regression of existing cysts. If the pa-tient wishes prophylaxis for the future, combination OCPs are a reasonable choice. Progestin-only pills are less effective in the suppression of ovulation, so they would be less effective in this patient.

B. Laparoscopic cystectomy is reserved for patients who are symptomatic for ovar-ian torsion. Such symptoms may include severe pain, fever, nausea, vomiting, and absent arterial and venous Doppler flow to the ovary on US.

C. Fine-needle aspiration of an ovarian cyst is often unsuccessful and is not indicated here.

D. Hospitalization and observation are indicated if a patient shows signs of intermittent torsion. This patient's symptoms are extremely mild, and torsion of a 2-cm cyst is unlikely. She should, however, be given precautionary information about returning for any signs or symptoms of ovarian torsion.

49. **A.** Treatment of Paget's disease consists of excision of all involved tissue with wide margins. Recurrence is more common than in vulvar intraepithelial lesions.

B. HPV infection has not been associated with Paget's disease of the vulva.

C. Paget's disease of the vulva is associated with a higher incidence of internal carcinoma, most commonly of the breast or colon.

D. Paget's disease is seen most commonly in postmenopausal women.

E. HSV-1 infection is most commonly associated with oral/labial lesions, but can also cause vulvar and vaginal lesions. HSV-2 infection is more commonly associated with genital tract lesions but can also cause oral lesions. Neither HSV type is associated with Paget's disease.

50. **A.** TOA or TOC most commonly results from PID; therefore, the same organisms are involved. Pathogenic organisms such as gonorrhea or chlamydia may be present and cultured from the cervix or the TOA at the time of surgical therapy. The most commonly found bacteria in TOAs are species of skin flora, gram-negative rods, and anaerobes such as *Streptococcus* spp., *Staphylococcus* spp., *Klebsiella* spp., *E. coli*, *Proteus* spp., *Bacteroides* spp., *Gardnerella vaginalis*, *Prevotella* spp., and *Peptostreptococcus*, among others. After 24 to 48 hours of IV antibiotics without improvement or if the patient develops signs of sepsis, drainage of the abscess should be performed. There are several modalities (e.g., laparotomy, laparoscopy, or imaging-guided needle drainage) to accomplish this to limit morbidity and mortality. Although TOA is most often associated with PID, it has been linked to other sources of pelvic infection, including diverticulitis, appendicitis, and pelvic surgeries and procedures.

B. As in the explanation for A, management is begun conservatively with antibiotics. Only if these measures fail to improve symptoms is drainage or surgery utilized.

C. TOA is most commonly a sequela of untreated PID, but it is also associated with ruptured appendicitis, pelvic surgery, hysterosalpingogram, and diverticulitis.

D. The most common feature in TOA is pain. In fact, more than 90% of patients report persistent low abdominal pain. Only 60% to 80% of patients have fever or leukocytosis. The patient invariably will have uterine tenderness, adnexal tenderness, and cervical motion tenderness. She may or may not have a palpable pelvic mass.

E. TOA is really a more severe subset of PID and carries with it all of the same risks of future infertility.

Setting 2: Office

Your office is in a primary care generalist group practice located in a physician office suite adjoining a suburban community hospital. Patients are usually seen by appointment. Most of the patients you see are from your own practice and are appearing for regular scheduled return visits, with some new patients as well. As in most group practices, you will often encounter a patient whose primary care is managed by one of your associates; reference may be made to the patient's medical records. You may do some telephone management, and you may have to respond to questions about articles in magazines and on television that will require interpretation. Complete laboratory and radiology services are available.

51. A 22-year-old sexually active woman comes into your office for a follow-up gynecological exam after her annual Pap smear 1 month ago showed morphology suggestive of cervical intraepithelial neoplasia type I (CIN I). On this visit, you perform a colposcopy with directed biopsies of small lesions seen in the transformation zone, as well as an endocervical curettage (ECC). Which of the following test results or historical information is an indication for further diagnosis and treatment via conization?

A. White epithelium is visible on colposcopy
B. Directed biopsies show changes consistent with CIN type III
C. The patient douches once per month
D. Punctation and mosaicism are seen on colposcopy
E. The patient is pregnant

52. A 52-year-old G_2P_2 woman presents with complaints of vaginal spotting, especially after intercourse, and a 15-pound weight loss in the last four months. On speculum exam, she is found to have a friable-appearing, cauliflower-shaped lesion in the transformation zone of her cervix. Subsequent biopsy of the lesion identifies it as squamous cell carcinoma. Which of the following would be considered a risk factor for cervical carcinoma in this patient?

A. She had her first child at age 31
B. She used a cervical cap as her primary mode of contraception for 30 years
C. She has a history of infection with HPV type 11
D. She has a 25 pack/year smoking history
E. She achieved menarche at the age of 15

53. A 29-year-old G_2P_1 woman presents at 27 weeks GA for a routine prenatal visit and third trimester labs. She has had an uncomplicated antenatal course up to this point. She weighs 82 kg now and her 3-year-old son's birthweight was 4500 g. The patient had a long labor with that delivery, which resulted in a cesarean section when she failed to dilate beyond 7 cm. She had an elevated glucose load test (GLT) in her last pregnancy of 147, but a normal 3-hour glucose tolerance test (GTT) of 80, 177, 151, 122. She has a maternal aunt who developed diabetes at age 57, but no other relatives with diabetes. In her history, which of the following is the biggest risk for her to have gestational diabetes (GD) in this pregnancy?

A. Previous elevated GLT
B. Prior macrosomic fetus
C. Aunt with type 2 diabetes
D. Prior gestational diabetes
E. Prior cesarean delivery

54. A 56-year-old postmenopausal woman is experiencing occasional vaginal bleeding and has had malodorous discharge, oliguria, and weight loss over several months. Vaginal exam reveals a cervical tumor involving much of the lower third of the vagina. On rectal exam, it is found that the tumor has obliterated the pouch of Douglas and extended all the way to the pelvic wall (Figure 54). A pelvic CT is remarkable for hydronephrosis of the left kidney, however, cytoscopy and proctoscopy are normal. The patient is diagnosed with cervical carcinoma. Based on these findings, what is her likely 5-year survival rate?

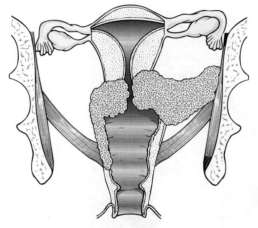

Figure 54 • Reproduced with permission from Callahan, T. Blueprints Obstetrics & Gynecology, 2nd ed. Blackwell Science, 2001: Fig. 26-2, p.212.

A. 4%
B. 40%
C. 72%
D. 88%
E. 95%

55. A 20-year-old woman presents to you with new onset of hair growth on her lower back, chest, and face. She reports no menstrual changes and no changes in her body shape or voice. She is not currently on any medications. Her FSH, LH, testosterone, and androgen precursor levels are all within the normal range. Exam reveals no pelvic mass, no changes in fat distribution, and no anatomical changes other than increased hair growth throughout her body. In the absence of a clear etiology, you diagnose this patient with constitutional (idiopathic) hirsutism. What is the best treatment option for her?

A. Danazol
B. Dehydroepiandrosterone (DHEA)
C. Cyclosporine
D. Spironolactone
E. Minocycline

56. A 28-year-old G$_0$ woman presents with a 7-month history of acne, deepening of her voice, and amenorrhea. She has never had menstrual irregularity in the past, and her past medical history is otherwise negative. Her exam is remarkable for a palpable pelvic mass and an enlarged clitoris. Labs show a negative pregnancy test; marked suppression of LH, FSH, and plasma androstenedione; and increased free testosterone levels. A pelvic US is obtained (Figure 56). You suspect a Sertoli-Leydig cell tumor, and promptly arrange for surgical removal. Which of the following statements is true regarding these tumors?

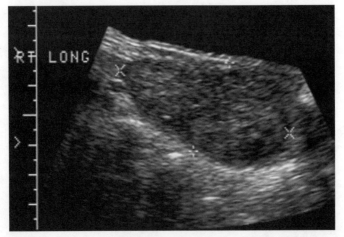

Figure 56 • Image provided by Departments of Radiology and Obstetrics & Gynecology, University of California, San Francisco.

    A. In the normal progression of disease, breast atrophy and amenorrhea precede clitoral hypertrophy
    B. With successful treatment of disease, there are no lasting sequelae
    C. Hirsutism is not a part of this syndrome
    D. The mortality rate for this tumor approaches 60%
    E. In the majority of cases, both ovaries are affected

57. A 19-year-old woman in a stable, monogamous relationship wishes to begin hormonal contraception. She has done some research and decided that she would prefer hormones over barrier methods because the latter are cumbersome and "ruin the mood." She does want to know more about specific hormone-based contraceptive methods, however, to help make her decision. Which of the following statements is most accurate regarding hormonal contraception?

    A. Combination OCPs exert their effect predominantly by use of estrogen to stimulate LH secretion
    B. Progestin-only pills allow more flexibility in dosing as compared to combination OCPs
    C. Progestin-only pills are contraindicated in lactating women
    D. The transdermal patch system has been shown to be twice as effective as combination OCPs
    E. Depo-Provera can safely be used in patients with epilepsy

58. A 19-year-old G_0 Caucasian woman presents to your office with complaints of lower abdominal and pelvic pain. She has experienced cyclic pain with her menses since the age of 14, but notes that over the past 12 to 15 months this pain has been increasing, leaving her unable to go to work for 2 to 3 days each month. For the past 2 months, she has had pain that occurs several times between her periods and lasts for several days. The patient has been sexually active since age 15, has used only condoms for contraception, and has never had any pelvic infections to her knowledge. She is currently in a monogamous sexual relationship, but has not been sexually active for the past month secondary to dyspareunia. She does note some relief of symptoms with 400 mg of ibuprofen. What is the next step in her diagnosis and treatment?

A. Laparoscopic resection of adhesions
B. Monophasic or continuous OCPs
C. Gonadotropin-releasing hormone (GnRH) analog therapy (Lupron)
D. Pain consult/psychiatry consult
E. Antibiotics

59. You are asked to see a couple regarding reversal of a sterilization procedure performed 4 years prior to their current visit. At that time, the couple had discussed a vasectomy, but the husband could not allay the many concerns he had regarding his ability to function sexually after the procedure. As a consequence, his wife decided to undergo a sterilization procedure, although she cannot recall which type. Now, however, the couple want another child. They cannot afford IVF, and feel that adoption would not be fulfilling because they believe that "one of the greatest joys of life is seeing each other in our children." Which of the following sterilization procedures, if done 4 years ago, would now offer the best chance of a successful reversal?

A. Falope ring
B. Pomeroy tubal ligation
C. Hulka clip
D. Electrocautery
E. Colpotomy

60. A 32-year-old G_1P_1 woman gave birth to a Down syndrome baby nearly 7 years ago. She now wants another child, but has concerns regarding this next pregnancy and her chances of having another child with Down syndrome. She therefore makes an appointment with a genetic counselor, who decides to screen her and her husband for a possible genetic predisposition to Down syndrome. The results of the karyotypes are as follows: Father: 46,XY; Mother: 45,XX, −21,−21, + t(21q;21q). What is the theoretical risk of their second-born child having Down syndrome?

A. 25%
B. 33%
C. 50%
D. 100%
E. Unable to determine from the information given

The next two questions (items 61 and 62) correspond to the following vignette.

A 34-year-old G_1P_0 woman at 17 weeks GA by LMP presents to your clinic for a follow-up appointment. At her last visit, she had an expanded AFP/maternal serum triple screen test. The results of the test came back with a low maternal serum alpha-fetoprotein (MSAFP), a low estriol level, and a high β-hCG. You are concerned, so you perform an US, which confirms that fetal size equals dates. Figure 61 is an image of the fetal abdomen.

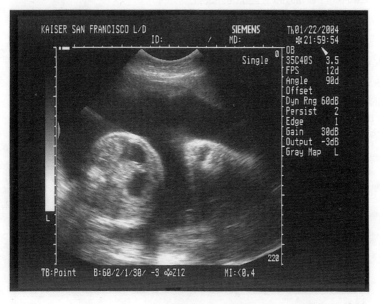

Figure 61 • Image courtesy of Susan H. Tran, Kaiser San Francisco Hospital, San Francisco, California.

61. These screening test results are most consistent with which of the following disorders/defects?

A. Edward's syndrome (trisomy 18)
B. Neural tube defects
C. Patau's syndrome (trisomy 13)
D. Down syndrome (trisomy 21)
E. Turner's syndrome (monosomy X)

62. What is the recommended next step in this patient's management?

A. Amniocentesis
B. Cordocentesis
C. CT scan of the abdomen
D. Chorionic villi sampling (CVS)
E. Nothing is indicated at this time; the fetus is not far enough along for accurate testing

End of set

---

63. A 23-year-old woman presents to your office with complaints of vulvar and vaginal pruritis. She became sexually active 2 weeks ago with a new partner and is concerned that these signs may be symptomatic of an STD. She complains of an increase in a white, clumpy discharge without odor. She notes no abdominal pain or fever. On physical exam, you note some erythematous punctate macular lesions bilaterally near the perineum, but no papular or vesicular lesions. On speculum exam, you observe a white discharge that has a negative whiff test; a KOH prepared slide reveals the image in Figure 63. What is the treatment of choice?

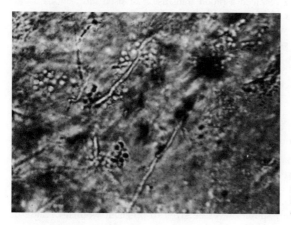

Figure 63 • Reproduced with permission from Crissey JT. Manual of Medical Mycology. Blackwell Science, 1995: 90.

A. Oral acyclovir
B. Topical acyclovir applied to the lesions
C. Oral metronidazole (Flagyl)
D. Vaginal metronidazole (Metro-gel)
E. Oral fluconazole (Diflucan)

64. A 26-year-old woman presents for her first prenatal visit after having a positive home pregnancy test 2 weeks ago. Her LMP began 7 weeks and 1 day ago. After taking a medical history, you perform a physical exam, perform a Pap smear, and take cultures for gonorrhea and chlamydia. In addition to these tests, which of the following would also be done at this visit?

    A. Triple screen of maternal serum alpha-fetoprotein, estriol, and β-hCG
    B. Diabetes mellitus screen
    C. Rh factor and antibody screen
    D. Group B *Streptococcus* culture
    E. Pelvic US

The next two questions (items 65 and 66) correspond to the following vignette.

A 32-year-old G$_4$P$_2$ woman sees you for her second prenatal visit at 17 weeks GA. She has two healthy children at home, both full-term vaginal deliveries following uncomplicated pregnancies. She agreed to an HIV test at her first visit, which is part of the universal screening that your clinic offers. Both the Western blot and ELISA are positive for HIV. The patient had never received a blood transfusion or used intravenous drugs. She is monogamous with her husband and believes their relationship to be mutually monogamous. He has no known exposures. She feels well in general and has no symptoms of opportunistic infections. Her viral load is undetectable. She is very concerned about passing the virus on to her baby, and has spent the last several days doing research on the Internet. Her understanding is that she will be started on antiretroviral therapy immediately and that she will need to have a cesarean delivery (although she desires vaginal delivery).

65. Which of the following corrections to her understanding best reflects the current standard of care for prevention of vertical transmission of HIV in the United States?

    A. If her viral load remains low, she will benefit from neither antiretroviral therapy nor cesarean section.
    B. Antiretroviral therapy does not need to be initiated until she is in labor, but cesarean section is indeed indicated.
    C. Antiretroviral therapy should never be given to pregnant women because of concerns about teratogenicity; cesarean section is indeed indicated.
    D. Antiretroviral therapy should be initiated now; if her viral count remains undetectable, a cesarean section is not necessarily indicated.
    E. Antiretroviral therapy should be initiated now; the fetus should be closely monitored with a scalp electrode as soon as the patient begins to labor, and cesarean section performed only for signs of distress.

66. This patient breastfed her previous two children, and is hoping to breastfeed this child as well. What is the most appropriate recommendation?

A. Her HIV status should have no bearing on breastfeeding choices, as the virus is not expressed in breast milk.

B. She should not breastfeed, because she is HIV positive.

C. She should not breastfeed, because the baby will require optimal nutrition to maximize immune system function, and this is best achieved with formula feeding.

D. Breastfeeding should be encouraged, as maternal immunoglobulins may protect the baby from infection.

E. Breastfeeding should be encouraged, as antiretroviral drugs given to the mother have been shown to be expressed in breast milk and provide a protective effect on the baby.

End of set

---

67. A 37-year-old G_1 woman presents at 26 weeks GA for a routine prenatal visit and review of her third trimester labs. She is dated by LMP, which was consistent with a normal 10-week US. Her antenatal course has been uncomplicated, although fatigue has forced her to limit her rehearsal schedule. Amniocentesis at 16 weeks GA (for advanced maternal age) showed a normal karyotype (46,XX). Last week her 50-g GLT was found to be elevated at 157. This morning she completed her 3-hour OGTT, which has just been reported to you as 86, 193, 173, 128. The patient denies personal or family history of diabetes. She is not obese and has no history of spontaneous abortions. As you begin to discuss the results of the OGTT, the patient becomes very tearful, explaining that she recently read in a magazine article that the risk of birth defects is increased in diabetic mothers. Which of the following is the most accurate way to counsel this patient regarding her concern?

A. The article is wrong; there is no connection between maternal diabetes and congenital anomalies

B. This patient probably has gestational diabetes, which, unlike overt (pregestational) diabetes, is not believed to carry an increased risk of fetal congenital anomalies

C. There is an increased risk of congenital anomalies in children of diabetic mothers, but her normal US at 10 weeks makes the risk of malformation very remote

D. There is an increased risk of congenital anomalies in children of diabetic mothers, but these are usually chromosomal in origin, so her normal amniocentesis result is very reassuring

E. The risk of birth defects is indeed increased, and oral hypoglycemic agents should be started to minimize this risk

68. A 13-year-old African American adolescent female presents to your office with complaints of lower abdominal pain that began 6 months ago. The pain lasts for 4 to 6 days and then decreases. For the last 2 months, the pain has lasted longer, and the patient now notes a fullness in her lower abdomen. She is not sexually active and has not begun menstruating yet. On physical exam, she is Tanner stage III. On abdominal exam, you note mild lower abdominal tenderness and a palpable fullness in her lower abdomen. On pelvic exam, you note that she has an intact hymenal ring and a foreshortened vaginal vault of only 2 cm above the hymenal ring. Figure 68 depicts her internal genitalia. What is the most likely diagnosis?

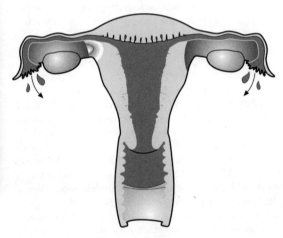

Figure 68

A. Testicular feminization
B. Imperforate hymen
C. Transverse vaginal septum
D. Labial fusion
E. Rudimentary uterine horn

69. A 32-year-old nonpregnant woman presents with complaints of minor changes to her body hair growth and changing voice beginning 2 months ago. She denies changes to her menses, and she is not currently taking any medications. Exam reveals mild increases in facial hair and low back hair growth, a slight deepening of her voice, and a blood pressure of 135/85. You suspect an endocrine disorder and begin a work-up. You find that her 24-hour free cortisol level is normal, but her free testosterone level is elevated at 220 ng/dL. A CT scan of her abdomen and pelvis is negative for masses. You decide to perform an ACTH stimulation test, which shows extremely elevated plasma levels of 11-deoxycorticosterone, but otherwise normal hormonal levels. Which of the following enzyme deficiencies could result in this finding?

A. 21-Hydroxylase
B. 11β-Hydroxylase
C. Aromatase
D. 3β-Hydroxysteroid dehydrogenase
E. 5α-Reductase

> The next two questions (items 70 and 71) correspond to the following vignette.

A 61-year-old G_0 woman presents for routine gynecologic exam. Her LMP was 7 years ago, and her last office visit was 2 years ago. She reports that she is in generally good health, but has felt vague abdominal discomfort for the last couple of months, which she attributes to stress resulting from adapting to a new format for the evening news. On bimanual exam, you note a unilateral, mobile adnexal mass on the left. The mass feels regular in shape.

70. Which one of the following is most concerning for malignancy, independently requiring further work-up?

    A. The mass is unilateral
    B. The mass is mobile
    C. The mass feels regular
    D. The cul-de-sac is smooth
    E. The patient is postmenopausal

71. A pelvic US is performed, which confirms a cystic mass measuring 4 cm on the left (Figure 71). Smooth internal and external contours are noted, as are multiple septations within the mass. No ascites are observed. Which of the following radiological findings is most suggestive of malignancy?

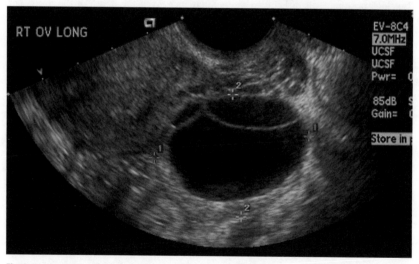

Figure 71 · Image provided by Departments of Radiology and Obstetrics & Gynecology, University of California, San Francisco.

    A. The mass is cystic
    B. The mass is smaller than 5 cm
    C. The mass has smooth contours
    D. The mass is septated
    E. No ascites are observed

End of set

72. A 49-year-old G_0 woman presents for routine annual exam. Her LMP was 3 years ago. She used OCPs for 7 years in her early twenties. At age 31, she had a 6-month course of clomiphene citrate for unexplained infertility, but later discovered that the basis of her inability to conceive was male factor. At age 33, no longer desiring pregnancy, she underwent bilateral tubal ligation. During today's visit, she expresses her concern about ovarian cancer because a friend was recently diagnosed with it. The patient has no family history of ovarian or breast cancer. Which of the following elements of this patient's history is most likely to increase her risk for ovarian cancer?

    A. Her age at menopause
    B. Her history of OCP use
    C. Her nulliparity
    D. Her tubal ligation
    E. Her history of clomiphene treatment

The next two questions (items 73 and 74) correspond to the following vignette.

A 35-year-old G_3P_3 who is 4 weeks postpartum presented 2 days ago with fever, chills, and left breast pain and erythema. She was diagnosed with mastitis and given outpatient oral antibiotics. Her systemic symptoms have greatly improved, but she continues to have mildly elevated temperatures to 100.0° F and persistent left breast pain. On physical exam, her left breast is not engorged but there is a deep, firm, 2 cm × 2 cm mass at the 3 o'clock position. It is difficult to assess fluctuance given the depth of the mass. The patient has continued to breastfeed from both breasts and has taken her antibiotics as prescribed since her prior visit. Her mother died of breast cancer at 49 years of age, and her sister is currently undergoing a work-up for a breast mass.

73. What should be the next step in evaluation?

    A. A core biopsy
    B. A breast US
    C. Incision and drainage in the OR
    D. A CT scan to evaluate for an abscess
    E. Reevaluation in 1 week

74. What is the most common pathogen in mastitis?

    A. *Staphylococcus aureus*
    B. *Staphylococcus epidermidis*
    C. *Pseudomonas aeruginosa*
    D. *Proprionobacterium acnes*
    E. *Lactococcal ductalis*

End of set

The next two questions (items 75 and 76) correspond to the following vignette.

A 26-year-old G_1P_1 had an uncomplicated normal, spontaneous vaginal delivery of a highly desired and healthy baby girl 4 days ago. Her husband calls the office stating that he is worried about his wife. Since coming home 2 days ago, she has experienced periods of crying for 1 to 2 hours at a time, followed by normal behavior, extreme irritability with him, and insomnia. He reports with concern that she forgot pots on the stove twice and burned the contents, which is very unusual for her because she is a professional chef. She has no known psychiatric history.

75. What is the most likely diagnosis?

A. Postpartum depression
B. Bipolar disorder
C. Postpartum blues
D. Malingering in the husband
E. Postpartum psychosis

76. A woman who had postpartum depression after the birth of her first child has what statistical risk for recurrence after her next birth?

A. 10%
B. 25%
C. 50%
D. 75%
E. 90%

End of set

77. A 26-year-old G_0 female had a routine Pap smear done at the time of a sexually transmitted infection screening visit. She was diagnosed with bacterial vaginosis and given a prescription for metronidazole vaginal gel at the appointment. Her Pap smear results are reported as HSIL. Her gonorrhea, chlamydia, syphilis, and HIV tests were all negative. What should be the next step in evaluating this patient?

A. Cold knife conization (CKC)
B. Repeat Pap smear every 4 months for 2 years until three consecutive smears are negative; do a colposcopy if and when a second smear is abnormal
C. Colposcopy and ECC
D. Cryotherapy
E. Treat her again for bacterial vaginosis and then repeat the Pap smear

78. A 37-year-old African American G_1P_0 woman at 41 weeks GA presents for her routine prenatal visit. Her pregnancy is complicated by a history of severe hyperemesis gravidarum until 16 weeks gestation that required two brief hospital stays for aggressive hydration. She has felt fine during the second half of her pregnancy. All of her routine prenatal labs have been within normal limits, and she had an amniocentesis performed at 15 weeks, which revealed a 46,XX fetus. She now presents 1 week after her due date wanting to know when she will deliver. On exam, her cervix is closed, but soft, and 50% effaced. She has a nonstress test (Figure 78). Given its appearance, you will reassure her that she is at lower risk for what condition over the ensuing week?

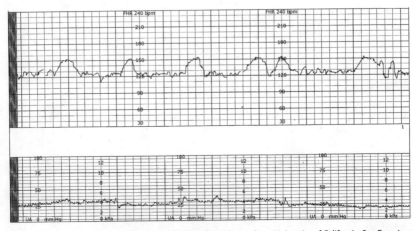

Figure 78 • Image provided by Department of Obstetrics & Gynecology, University of California, San Francisco.

A. Gestational diabetes (GD)
B. Intrauterine fetal demise (IUFD)
C. Meconium in the amniotic fluid
D. Macrosomia
E. Preeclampsia

79. A 27-year-old attorney presents to your gynecologic clinic for an annual exam. She has not had an exam for 3 years, but has not experienced any problems prior to her current visit. She presents because she is interested in birth control, as she is now in a monogamous sexual relationship. As part of this routine exam, you perform a Pap smear, test for gonorrhea and chlamydia, and start the patient on a monophasic oral contraceptive pill. The Pap smear returns with a result of LSIL/CIN I. You meet with the patient 2 weeks later to discuss the ramifications of this finding. You tell her the following in your discussion:

A. With CIN I, the average length of time to the development of cervical cancer is 3 to 4 years
B. 10% of CIN I lesions resolve spontaneously
C. The next step in management is cryotherapy
D. Cervical dysplasia is highly associated with HPV subtypes 16 and 18
E. The next step in management is laser therapy

80. A 66-year-old African American woman presents to the office complaining of external vaginal dryness and itching for the last 3 months. She suspected a yeast infection and tried two over-the-counter antifungal creams with no relief. She has also tried vinegar douches with no relief. She is not sexually active, and her LMP was 12 years ago. She does not take HRT. On exam, you find moderate vaginal mucosal atrophy and a small (less than 1 cm), white-based, nontender ulcer on the inferior left labia majus. No exophytic lesions are noted. Which of the following steps should you take?

A. Prescribe a topical estrogen cream and reevaluate in 3 weeks
B. Prescribe a topical steroid cream and reevaluate in 3 weeks
C. Perform a wide local excision in the office
D. Perform a punch biopsy
E. Reassure her that vulvar pruritis is normal in postmenopausal women and offer her HRT

81. A 67-year-old female patient of yours notes an abnormal vaginal discharge on and off for longer than 6 months. Each time she thought it was a yeast infection like those she experienced as a young woman and used an over-the-counter antifungal vaginal cream with minimal relief. She came to your office on this occasion because she noticed a bloody tinge to the discharge. On exam, you note a foul-smelling discharge and a large mucosal abnormality on the upper-left vaginal wall. You take a biopsy and have a high suspicion for vaginal carcinoma. Where does squamous cell carcinoma of the vagina most commonly occur?

A. At the introitus
B. In the upper one-third of the vagina
C. In the lower two-thirds of the vagina
D. On the labia majora
E. Equally in all vaginal areas

The next two questions (items 82 and 83) correspond to the following vignette.

A non–sexually active 42-year-old woman was found to have a large mass in the mucosa of the posterior fornix on pelvic exam as part of a work-up for recurrent UTIs. On bimanual exam, the mass was felt to extend to the left pelvic sidewall. A biopsy was done and returned as "invasive squamous cell carcinoma with lymphatic invasion."

82. Which of the following lymph nodes would you first expect to be positive?

   A. None; vaginal cancer spreads hematogenously
   B. Femoral triangle nodes
   C. Internal and common iliac nodes
   D. Supraclavicular
   E. Posterior cervical

83. Given the above information, what stage is this woman's disease?

   A. Stage I
   B. Stage II
   C. Stage III or IV
   D. Stage V
   E. Unable to assign until tissue borders are evaluated on the pathologic specimen

End of set

---

84. A 27-year-old G_1P_1 presents to your office for preconception counseling. Her prior delivery was significant for a primary low transverse cesarean section for fetal intolerance of labor. She desires a trial of labor for her subsequent pregnancy. You counsel her that:

   A. Her risk of uterine rupture is 5% to 10%
   B. Management of uterine rupture includes expectant management and laparoscopy
   C. Risk of uterine rupture is increased by induction of labor
   D. Fetal mortality rate is greater than 50% should uterine rupture occur
   E. Use of oxytocin during labor may decrease her risk for uterine rupture

85. A 36-year-old G_1P_0 at 42 0/7 weeks GA presents for a routine prenatal appointment followed by antenatal testing (nonstress test and amniotic fluid index). Her NST is reactive and her amniotic fluid index is 6. On exam, her cervix is found to be favorable with a Bishop's score of 6. She declines your recommendation to proceed with post-term labor induction. In counseling the patient, you tell her that post-term pregnancy (more than 42 weeks GA) includes an increased risk of:

   A. Polyhydramnios
   B. Meconium aspiration
   C. Rh sensitization
   D. Low birthweight
   E. Respiratory distress syndrome

86. A 32-year-old G$_2$P$_1$ with a twin pregnancy at 26 4/7 weeks GA presents for her prenatal visit. She is noted to have size greater than dates on physical exam and is sent for a formal US for further evaluation. The US is notable for polyhydramnios of one twin and oligohydramnios and growth restriction of the other twin. In addition, the image in Figure 86 is obtained of the twin with polyhydramnios. What is the most likely diagnosis?

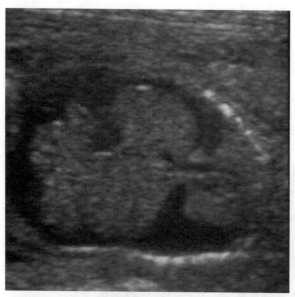

Figure 86 • Image provided by Departments of Radiology and Obstetrics & Gynecology, University of California, San Francisco.

A. Twin–twin transfusion syndrome
B. Rh incompatibility
C. "Siamese" twinning
D. Normal variant of monozygotic twinning
E. Congenital rubella syndrome

87. An 18-year-old woman presents for her annual exam requesting OCPs and complaining of 3 months of amenorrhea. She experienced menarche at age 12 and had regular menses every 28 days until the last 3 months. She became sexually active at age 16 and is currently monogamous with her boyfriend of 4 months. She is completing her freshman year as a premedical student and is a member of the freshman track team. Despite her rigorous exercise regimen, she notes a 5 lb weight gain over the past 4 months. What is the most likely cause of secondary amenorrhea in this patient?

A. Kallmann's syndrome
B. Hypothyroidism
C. Pregnancy
D. Exercise
E. Stress

88. A 36-year-old G_2P_1 Asian woman presents for her fourth prenatal visit at 17 weeks GA. She had some nausea and vomiting in the first trimester that resolved by 14 weeks gestation; otherwise, she has had an entirely uncomplicated pregnancy. At her last appointment at 15 weeks gestation, she underwent screening for maternal serum alpha-fetoprotein (MSAFP). The result returned 2 days ago with a value that is 4.5 multiples of the median (MoMs). Which of the following is the most unlikely etiology of this abnormal result?

A. Anencephaly
B. Twin gestation
C. Gastroschisis
D. Trisomy 18
E. She is actually 19 weeks GA

89. A 26-year-old woman with no significant past medical history presents to you for evaluation after having two miscarriages in the past 2 years. During an office US, you note a bicornuate uterus (Figure 89). To evaluate further, you order a hysterosalpingogram. Which of the following is associated with a bicornuate uterus?

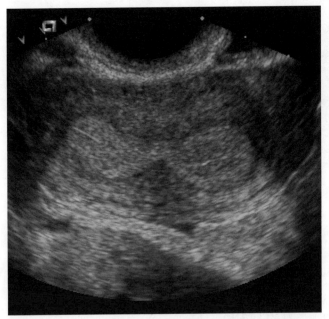

Figure 89 • Image provided by Departments of Radiology and Obstetrics & Gynecology, University of California, San Francisco.

A. Endometriosis
B. Uterine cancer
C. Premature labor
D. Urinary tract infections
E. Fetal anomalies

90. A 33-year-old G_3P_0 visits your office for consultation regarding her pregnancy history of three consecutive pregnancy losses at 10, 13, and 11 weeks of gestation. She and her partner are interested in an evaluation for the etiology of the losses. You explain that possible causes may include thrombophilia, genetic abnormalities in one or both of the partners, uterine cavity abnormalities, and endocrine or immune system dysfunction. Which of the following choices correctly matches a cause with the best treatment for the losses?

A. Septate uterus—surgery
B. Balanced translocation—Clomid with intrauterine insemination
C. Antiphospholipid antibody syndrome—corticosteroids
D. Hyperprolactinemia—corticosteroids
E. Group B *Streptococcus*—antibiotics

91. You are seeing a 26-year-old woman in her second trimester of pregnancy who has a history of a prior cesarean delivery. She inquires about a trial of labor (TOL) to achieve a vaginal birth after cesarean section (VBAC). Which of the following is a contraindication to TOL in this setting?

A. History of prior cesarean section being 7 months ago
B. History of cesarean section for breech
C. History of Kerr (low transverse) incision with a "T" extension into the active segment
D. History of Kronig (low vertical) incision
E. History of successful VBAC complicated by postpartum hemorrhage

92. A 33-year-old G_3P_2 Caucasian woman at 14 weeks GA presents for her second prenatal visit. She has had two prior uncomplicated births: a daughter, age 7, and a son, age 3. Her first trimester prenatal labs done at 11 weeks of gestation revealed that she is Rh-negative and has an anti-D antibody titer of 1:4. She found out that she was Rh-negative in her first pregnancy; at birth, her daughter was also Rh-negative. The patient's last pregnancy was uncomplicated, and she had a negative antibody titer throughout. Her son was Rh-positive. The patient received RhoGAM (anti-D immune globulin) in her last two pregnancies at 28 weeks, but not after delivery in either one. Her Caucasian husband is the father of all of her pregnancies. Given that the rate of Rh-negative individuals is 16% among Caucasians, which of the following statements is true regarding this patient?

A. Her husband has a 48% chance of being heterozygous
B. There is a possibility that her husband is Rh-negative
C. The probability that this fetus is Rh-negative is 0.5
D. A dose of RhoGAM in this pregnancy will be protective
E. This patient will need serial amniocentesis in this pregnancy if the fetus is Rh-positive

93. An obese 78-year-old G_0 woman presents to your office with complaints of heavy vaginal spotting for the last 2 weeks. She is concerned because her periods stopped 22 years ago. She reports an uneventful transition to menopause after a long history of irregular periods. She tells you that she has never liked taking pills and did not use OCPs or HRT. What is the best way to care for this patient?

A. US
B. Reassurance and a follow-up appointment in 2 weeks
C. Endometrial biopsy
D. Pap smear
E. D&C

94. You are a urogynecologist evaluating a 67-year-old female for urinary stress incontinence. Your patient reports that she wears a large panty shield at all times because of her fear of leaking urine. She tells you she has been wearing the pads for 1 year and now is concerned that the pads are causing an allergic reaction because she has been suffering from severe vulvar itching over the last 2 months. Upon exam, you note a raised white lesion. Your clinical suspicion is that this lesion is most likely which of the following?

    A. Contact dermatitis
    B. Yeast infection
    C. Lichen simplex chronicus
    D. Lichen sclerosus et atrophicus
    E. Vulvar cancer

95. A 27-year-old G_3P_2 woman presents to your office at 19 weeks GA after just having had her obstetric US. You call the ultrasonologist for the results and find that the fetus had a normal US except for bilateral choroid plexus cysts (Figure 95). The patient's pregnancy has been uncomplicated to this point, and her second trimester serum screening results returned with lower than age-related risks of both trisomies 21 and 18. You prepare to tell her that this finding has been associated with which of the following?

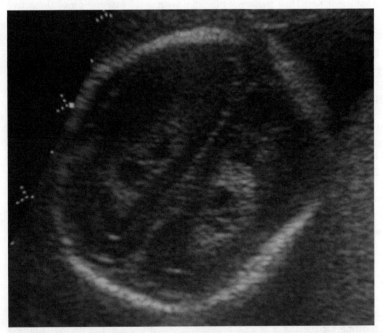

Figure 95 • Image provided by Departments of Radiology and Obstetrics & Gynecology, University of California, San Francisco.

    A. Trisomy 18
    B. Anencephaly
    C. Neural tube defects (NTDs)
    D. Developmental delay
    E. Turner's syndrome

96. A 22-year-old G_0 Korean woman presents with complaints of increased body and facial hair. She has noticed increased hair growth on her upper lip, chin, upper back, and lower abdomen for about 5 years. She denies deepening of her voice, balding, or enlargement of her clitoris. None of the other women in her family has any of these symptoms, and she feels quite self-conscious as a result. The patient underwent menarche at age 13, has irregular menses every 25 to 45 days, and has never been sexually active. On physical exam, she is 5 ft 4 in. tall and weighs 154 lb. She has some generalized acne on her face and back in addition to acanthosis nigricans. There are a few terminal hairs on her back as well as some stubble on her cheeks and upper lip. Her escutcheon is diamond-shaped. Lab tests show the following results: normal 17-α-hydroxyprogesterone, normal testosterone, a luteinizing hormone to follicle-stimulating hormone ratio (LH:FSH) of 4, normal DHEA-S, and normal function of 5-α-reductase. What is the most likely diagnosis?

A. Sertoli-Leydig cell tumor
B. Congenital adrenal hyperplasia (CAH)
C. Testicular feminization
D. Germ cell tumor
E. Polycystic ovarian syndrome (PCOS)

97. A 32-year-old G_2P_2 woman presents complaining of vaginal fullness and occasional vaginal pain and urinary urgency. She denies urinary or fecal incontinence. Her symptoms began shortly after the birth of her second child 3 months ago and worsen when she exercises. Her delivery was vaginal and uncomplicated, and the baby weighed 7 lb 4 oz. The patient is not breastfeeding. A pelvic exam reveals a first-degree cystocele (Figure 97), but the remainder of the exam is unremarkable. Urinary and cervical cultures are negative, and her postpartum Pap smear was negative. What is the most appropriate next step?

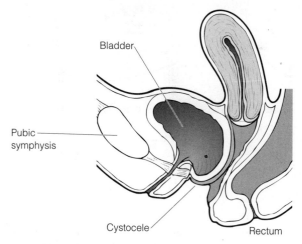

Bladder

Pubic symphysis

Cystocele

Rectum

Figure 97

A. Estrogen therapy
B. Anterior repair
C. Kegel exercises
D. Colpocleisis
E. Pessary

98. A 63-year-old woman presents with complaints of leaking urine. She started noticing occasional leakage about 6 months ago, occurring approximately once or twice a week during physical activity (hiking or yoga). Over the past month, however, she has noted an increase in frequency, leaking small amounts of urine several times a day. The patient developed an upper respiratory infection 2 weeks ago and noticed that she leaked urine whenever she coughed. She does not notice any leakage while she sleeps or while she is seated, but will have a small leak when she rises from sitting. She denies dysuria or inability to control micturition if she feels a urinary urge. Other past medical history reveals that she is a G_5P_4 with four vaginal deliveries. She went through menopause at age 51 and is not currently taking HRT. On physical exam, you note mild uterine descensus and a grade I cystocele. A Q-tip test (Figure 98) is positive with an angle change from $10°$ to approximately $45°$. You tell her she most likely has:

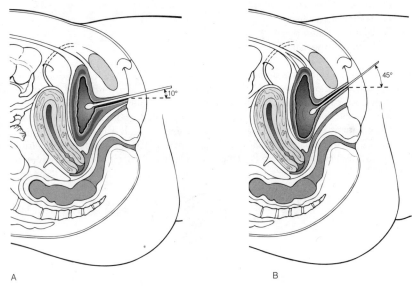

A   B

Figure 98 • Reproduced with permission from Callahan T. Blueprints Obstetrics & Gynecology. 3rd ed. Blackwell, 2004: Fig. 19-4B, p. 171.

    A. Stress incontinence
    B. Urge incontinence
    C. Detrusor instability
    D. Total incontinence
    E. Overflow incontinence

99. A 24-year-old G_2P_0 woman presents at 18 weeks GA for her routine obstetric US. She notes no fevers, chills, changes in bowel or urinary function, or abdominal pain. She has had an uncomplicated pregnancy up to this point and had an elective termination of her last pregnancy at 12 weeks. The US is performed, and the resulting image of the cervix and vagina is shown in Figure 99. A sterile speculum exam is performed and reveals no evidence of ruptured membranes, trichomoniasis, or bacterial vaginosis. At this point, her management could include which of the following?

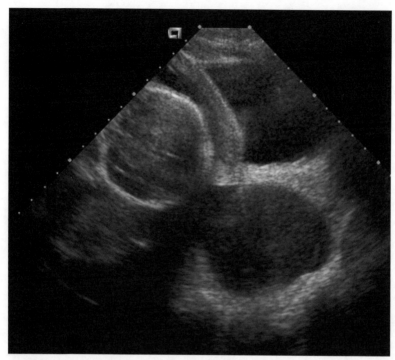

Figure 99 • Image provided by Departments of Radiology and Obstetrics & Gynecology, University of California, San Francisco.

A. Oral metronidazole (Flagyl)
B. Termination of pregnancy
C. Vaginal clindamycin (Cleocin)
D. Tocolysis with magnesium sulfate
E. Betamethasone for fetal lung maturity

100. A 19-year-old G_1P_0 woman at 28 weeks GA by LMP is Rh-negative, while her husband is Rh-positive. When you perform an antibody screen of the mother for Rh sensitivity, you find that she is unsensitized (i.e., she does not possess antibodies to Rh factor). What is the appropriate next step in the management of this patient?

A. Schedule an amniocentesis
B. Recheck the father's Rh status, as this result is incompatible with the mother's current antibody status
C. Counsel the couple about the high likelihood that this baby will be born with a hemolytic anemia
D. Administer 300 μg of RhoGAM immediately
E. No intervention other than close monitoring is indicated at this time

Answer Key

51.	B	68.	C	85.	B
52.	D	69.	B	86.	A
53.	B	70.	E	87.	C
54.	B	71.	D	88.	D
55.	D	72.	C	89.	C
56.	A	73.	B	90.	A
57.	E	74.	A	91.	C
58.	B	75.	C	92.	C
59.	C	76.	B	93.	C
60.	D	77.	C	94.	C
61.	D	78.	B	95.	A
62.	A	79.	D	96.	E
63.	E	80.	D	97.	C
64.	C	81.	B	98.	A
65.	D	82.	C	99.	B
66.	B	83.	C	100.	D
67.	B	84.	C		

51. **B.** Conization (also called cone biopsy) is a procedure in which a cone-shaped piece of cervical tissue is removed for analysis. It can be performed using either a scalpel, known as a cold knife cone, or an electrocautery device. The specimen taken includes the entire squamocolumnar junction (SCJ), any visible ectocervical lesions, and a portion of the endocervical canal. One indication for this procedure is a two-step discrepancy between Pap smear and subsequent guided biopsies, as seen in this case where the Pap smear shows CIN I and the biopsies show CIN III. Such a large difference warrants further testing, and a cone biopsy aids in resolving this discrepancy. A second indication for conization is an unsatisfactory colposcopy, where either the SCJ or margins of abnormal areas cannot be visualized in their entirety. In this situation, conization allows for better visualization of both areas. A positive ECC showing signs of dysplasia is a third indication for conization. ECC provides cytologic information for areas located farther inside the cervical canal. Because ECC does not provide any information on tissue orientation, however, it is impossible to determine the degree of dysplasia present in these samples. Conization provides the means for further analysis. Of note, conization can also be used as a therapeutic measure, usually to remove portions of the cervix that contain high-grade dysplastic changes or frank cervical carcinoma in situ.

A. Colposcopy helps to better visualize the TZ, where 95% of cervical cellular changes are found. The cervix is first prepped with acetic acid to dehydrate cells and precipitate proteins in the nucleus. Because neoplastic cells contain higher nuclear:cytoplasm ratios, they appear whiter than the surrounding epithelium. This white epithelium helps to guide biopsies but does not indicate the need for further work-up or treatment. Other signs of neoplasia on colposcopy include abnormal vasculature and visible punctate lesions.

C. While douching is known to predispose a woman to bacterial vaginosis and trichomoniasis by raising the pH in the vagina, it is not linked to cervical dysplasia or cancer.

D. Punctation and mosaicism are visual signs of dysplastic cells and deserve colposcopic-directed biopsy. Only if those biopsy results are consistent with more aggressive disease does the patient need to progress to conization.

E. Pregnancy is an absolute contraindication to conization because there is significant risk for the development of cervical incompetence and premature delivery.

52. **D.** Smoking is believed to increase the risk for cervical cancer by decreasing the body's ability to clear cancer-causing HPV (see the explanation for C) from the body. Other major risk factors for cervical cancer include early age at first coitus (especially within 1 year of menarche), multiple sexual partners, young age at first pregnancy, high parity, low SES, and divorce.

A. See the explanation for D.

B. While cervical caps have been linked to cervicitis, inflammation, and toxic shock syndrome, they play no role in the pathogenesis of cervical cancer.

C. HPV is the principal causative agent of cervical cancer. Leading theories link HPV with dysplasia, with evidence suggesting that it may induce epithelial cells to undergo abnormal maturation processes and unchecked mitosis. However, only certain types of HPV are linked to cancer and/or dysplasia—namely, 16, 18, 31, 33, 35, 39, 45, 51, 52, 56, and 58. HPV type 11, as well as type 6, is a proven cause of condyloma acuminata (venereal warts), but not cervical cancer.

E. Menarche, regardless of age, is not correlated with cervical cancer.

53. | **B.** GD is a phenomenon seen in pregnancy related to diminished ability to metabolize and utilize carbohydrates efficiently. It is likely a product of a combination of factors, including a baseline mild carbohydrate intolerance combined with anti-insulin agents synthesized by the placenta (e.g., human placental lactogen, HPL) that increase throughout the second and third trimesters of pregnancy. GD is classified into two types: A1 (diet controlled) and A2 (medication dependent). GD has been associated with increased birthweight and birth injury, but not with fetal anomalies as has pregestational diabetes. It is also associated with increased likelihood of maternal type 2 diabetes in the future. This patient's biggest risk factor for developing GD is history of a prior macrosomic fetus. Other risk factors include prior GD, first-degree relative with diabetes, and Latina, South Pacific Islander, or Native American ethnicity.

A. Because the GLT is a screening test and has many false-positive results, an elevated GLT in a prior pregnancy has not been shown to increase risk of diabetes in a subsequent pregnancy.

C. While a history of affected second-degree relatives has not been well studied as a risk factor, it seems likely that there is a mild association with the development of GD. However, this correlation is not as strong as that noted with the other risk factors listed in the explanation for B.

D. The patient did not have GD in her last pregnancy. Otherwise, that would be the major risk factor.

E. Prior cesarean section has not been associated with GD in epidemiologic studies.

54. | **B.** This patient presents with Stage IIIB cervical cancer. Hallmarks include involvement of the lower one-third of the vagina, extension to the pelvic wall, and renal dysfunction that is not otherwise explained. The 5-year survival rate in general for Stage III cancer ranges from 36% to 44%. Stage I cancer is preclinical. It is confined to the cervix with minimal stromal invasion and microscopic lesions not larger than 7 mm across and 5 mm deep. The 5-year survival rate for Stage I cancer ranges from 85% to 100%. Stage II cancer extends beyond the cervix, but has not reached the pelvic wall. It may involve the vagina, but has not yet extended to the lower one-third. The 5-year survival rate for Stage II cancer ranges from 68% to 80%. Stage IV cancer has extended beyond the true pelvis to adjacent organs (bladder/rectum) or distant sites. Most commonly affected organs include lung, liver, and bone. Overall 5-year survival rates are dismal—only 2% to 15%.

A, C, D, E. See the explanation for B.

55. **D.** Spironolactone is traditionally used as a diuretic agent due to its effect on aldosterone receptors. However, this drug also decreases production of testosterone and works in hair follicles to decrease local binding of dihydrotestosterone (DHT, a potent stimulator of hair growth) to androgen receptors via competitive inhibition, leading to resolution of abnormal hair growth.

A. Danazol is a weak androgenic drug used for treatment of endometriosis. It can actually cause hirsutism and other virilizing changes in some women. It is not an appropriate therapy for constitutional hirsutism.

B. DHEA is an important precursor of androstenedione and testosterone. It is not appropriate therapy for hirsutism.

C. Cyclosporine is an immunosuppressive agent used to treat inflammatory bowel disease, aplastic anemia, psoriasis, and various types of cancers. It is not known to decrease androgenic concentrations in hair follicles but has been shown to cause hirsutism in some patients.

E. Minocycline is a tetracycline-class antibiotic used primarily for the treatment of acne vulgaris. Common side effects include staining of teeth; hyperpigmentation of skin, nails, conjunctiva, tongue, and internal organs; and other rare autoimmune disorders. However, this agent does not affect hair growth.

56. **A.** Sertoli-Leydig cell tumor is a rare ovarian neoplasm that accounts for less than 0.5% of all ovarian tumors. Peak incidence is between 20 and 40 years of age. Generally, a characteristic clinical course is observed, in which defeminizing changes such as amenorrhea, breast atrophy, and loss of subcutaneous fat precede the masculinizing changes of clitoral hypertrophy, hirsutism, and deepening voice. Progression is rapid, however, with most of these changes occurring within 6 months. Treatment is prompt surgical removal of the tumor; the 10-year survival rate for this type of cancer exceeds 90%.

B. Some of the masculinizing changes such as clitoral enlargement and terminal hair growth do not regress after the tumor has been removed. However, temporal balding, menstrual changes, female body habitus, and future hair growth patterns do return to normal.

C. See the explanation for A. Hirsutism is a major symptom of this disorder.

D. See the explanation for A. This is generally a low-grade, highly curable disease.

E. Bilateral ovarian involvement is relatively rare, though when this diagnosis is made it is imperative that the contralateral ovary be inspected for gross changes.

57. **E.** Depo-Provera does not interfere with the metabolism or action of antiseizure medications, and thus is safe for use in patients with epilepsy. Furthermore, progesterone has been associated with diminished seizure activity. Combination OCPs, on the other hand, are relatively contraindicated due to interference by most antiseizure medications on combination OCP metabolism and efficacy.

A. Combination OCPs exert their effect mostly by use of progestins to block LH secretion, thereby preventing ovulation. Progestins also serve to thicken cervical mucus, thereby inhibiting sperm passage and decreasing fallopian tube peristalsis, which interferes with zygote transport and implantation. The estrogenic component is important in blocking FSH secretion, which prevents the development of a dominant ovarian follicle. When used in combination, these hormones effect atrophic changes in the uterine lining, thereby hindering implantation.

B. Progestin-only OCPs exert essentially the same effects as do the progestin components of combination OCPs. However, the low doses of progestin are not as effective in preventing ovulation, which can happen as much as 40% of the time. In addition, the low doses of progestin necessitate taking progestin-only OCPs at almost the same time every day to reduce the risk of failure, making them inherently less flexible.

C. Progestin-only OCPs have no effect on the contents or production of breast milk, and there is no evidence of nursing infants being adversely affected by progestin-only OCPs. Lactating women actually have a lower failure rate with progestin-only OCPs compared to the general population, however, because high circulating prolactin levels further suppress ovulation.

D. Numerous studies have confirmed the equal efficacy of the transdermal patch with traditional combination OCPs.

58. | **B.** This patient gives an excellent history for endometriosis. It is likely she has endometrial implants in her pelvis that undergo the same cycle as her endometrium and become inflamed each month with her menses. Over time, these implants can become scarred, cause adhesions, and lead to pain that is intermenstrual and eventually continuous. This pain can become quite debilitating, leading to change in work, school, and social habits. The first step in the treatment of endometriosis involves the administration of OCPs and NSAIDs. If the patient notes relief from pain except during menses, the OCPs can be given continuously with just one or two withdrawal bleeds per year.

A. Laparoscopy in the setting of endometriosis and pelvic pain in general should be used after the patient has failed medical treatment. Laparoscopy is the gold standard for diagnosis of endometriosis, allowing biopsy for pathological confirmation and resection of endometrial implants. Resection of the implants and lysis of adhesions have also been shown to give symptomatic relief. This relief, however, is rarely permanent.

C. The GnRH analog Lupron (leuprolide) is used in severe cases of endometriosis. It causes ovarian suppression and effectively produces a menopausal-like state. While this can give symptomatic relief, it can also lead to other problems due to the prolonged hypoestrogenic state, such as osteoporosis. Any patient undergoing GnRH therapy should have a bone density scan at baseline and be followed during treatment.

D. Consultation with the pain and psychiatry services can be an important aspect of management. However, this can often lead to alienation of the patient, who may infer that you think her pain is "in her head." Thus it is better to provide medical therapy first and form a therapeutic bond with the patient. If the medical therapy fails, then you should consider these consults prior to surgery.

E. Although both chronic PID and endometritis are causes of chronic pain treatable with antibiotics, this patient's story is not consistent with either diagnosis. Cultures should be taken at the initial exam to rule out PID.

59. | **C.** This procedure involves placing a plastic clip (Figure 59a) similar to a staple on the isthmus of the tube to occlude passage of ova. It is the most easily reversed procedure (success rates are as high as 50% to 75%), because only a very small portion of the tubes is damaged during the procedure. It also carries the highest failure rate for this reason—as high as 1%.

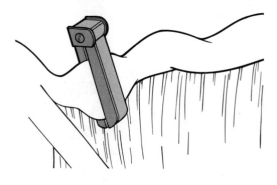

Figure 59a · Reproduced with permission from Callahan T. Blueprints Obstetrics & Gynecology. 3rd ed. Blackwell, 2004: Fig. 24-11, p. 221.

A. The Falope ring (Figure 59b) is similar to the Hulka clip, except that it involves placement of a single ring around two adjacent portions of the tube. It has a slightly lower failure rate, and a lower rate of successful reversal, than the clip.

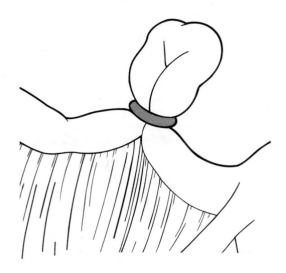

Figure 59b · Reproduced with permission from Callahan T. Blueprints Obstetrics & Gynecology. 3rd ed. Blackwell, 2004: Fig. 24-10, p. 221.

B. This is the most commonly used of the ligation techniques, whereby the proximal and distal borders of the middle third of the tube are ligated and the section of tube in between is removed (Figure 59c). The ends then seal closed over time. This procedure presents a much more difficult reversal task, and success rates hover near 25% to 50%.

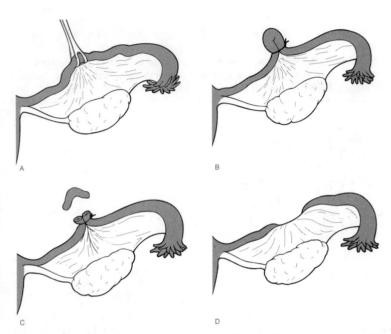

Figure 59c • Reproduced with permission from Callahan T. Blueprints Obstetrics & Gynecology. 3rd ed. Blackwell, 2004: Fig. 24–12 A–D, p. 222.

D. Electrocautery involves electrical ligation of portions of the tube using coagulation forceps. It is fast and very reliable, and the most difficult procedure to reverse because of the extensive damage done to the tube. There is also a higher risk of damage to adjacent organs during the procedure.

E. Colpotomy describes the surgical approach through the vagina taken to sterilize a patient, and is not a procedure in itself. Any of the laparoscopic or laparotomy procedures can be performed via this approach.

60. | **D.** The mother's karyotype represents a balanced Robertsonian translocation, in which her two copies of chromosome 21 (which are acrocentric) have lost their very short p sections and subsequently joined their q sections into one chromosome. Because karyotypes are done on cultured lymphocytes from peripheral blood, this represents the karyotype of all her cells, including germ cells. Therefore, when her germ cells undergo meiosis, 50% of them will have two copies of chromosome 21 (joined as a single chromosome), while the other 50% will have no copies of chromosome 21. When these gametes subsequently join with a normal paternal gamete containing one copy of chromosome 21, half of the resulting embryos will be trisomic for 21, and the other half will be monosomic for 21. One would conclude, then, that this couple's chance of having a Down syndrome baby is 50%. However, because monosomy 21 is incompatible with life and all such embryos are spontaneously aborted, all live births will be trisomy 21 births, leaving this couple with a 100% chance that their next baby will have Down syndrome.

A, B, C, E. See the explanation for D.

61. **D.** The combined pattern of elevated β-hCG, low MSAFP, and low estriol is concerning for Down syndrome. However, many factors contribute to the interpretation of these results, including maternal age, weight, ethnicity, mother's diabetic status, and multiple gestations. A likelihood of Down syndrome is then determined based on these factors. Note that the vast majority of mothers with a positive triple screen will deliver normal, healthy infants. In addition to the triple screen abnormalities, the finding on US of a likely pyloric stenosis or duodenal atresia as indicated by the "double-bubble" sign increases the likelihood of Down syndrome.

A. Edward's syndrome (trisomy 18) is similar to Down syndrome, except that symptoms are much more severe. Edward's syndrome infants usually do not survive more than a few days after birth, and only 10% will live 1 year. They present with severe mental retardation and defects in many organ systems. This is usually represented by low estriol (similar to Down syndrome) and low β-hCG (opposite of Down syndrome) levels.

B. Neural tube defects include such disorders as spina bifida, meningocele, and anencephaly. Generally, these abnormalities are indicated by an elevated MSAFP (opposite of Down syndrome), elevated amniotic AFP, and, in the case of anencephaly, a low β-hCG (also opposite of Down syndrome). Depending on severity, some types of neural tube defects can be corrected surgically.

C. Trisomy 13 (Patau's syndrome) is the least common and most severe of the autosomal trisomies. It is characterized by severe mental retardation, neurologic abnormalities including holoprosencephaly (the brain does not divide into distinct hemispheres), cardiac and other organic structural defects, and death within 3 days. This disorder is not associated with any findings on the triple screen.

E. Turner's syndrome presents as a girl with short stature, webbed neck, amenorrhea, and absence of secondary sex characteristics. Generally, this disorder is not diagnosed until puberty, when these findings become much more noticeable. As with trisomy 13, there is no association between Turner's syndrome and the triple screen.

62. **A.** The combination of results is associated with a higher risk of a fetus with Down syndrome. An abnormal result can also be seen with a pregnancy that is earlier than predicted by LMP. However, this outcome is less likely in this case because the US confirmed that the fetus's GA is the same as its calculated age by LMP. To evaluate for Down syndrome, a formal karyotype of the fetus is needed. This can be accomplished by using either amniocentesis (a process by which amniotic fluid is drawn via a needle using US guidance), cordocentesis, or chorionic villi sampling. Amniocentesis is generally performed at or around 15 weeks, making it the most appropriate choice in this case.

B. Cordocentesis is done by inserting a spinal needle, via US guidance, into an umbilical cord vessel to draw blood for analysis. It has a much higher complication rate than amniocentesis and is reserved for situations where rapid diagnosis is important.

C. A CT scan would not provide any additional information.

D. CVS involves sampling of chorionic villi taken either through the cervix or through the abdomen. This procedure is generally done at 9 to 12 weeks GA.

E. See the explanation for A.

63. | **E.** The patient has vulvovaginal candidiasis, which presents with pruritis and a white discharge, and which may have an instigator such as a change in sexual habits, undergarments, or a course of antibiotics. Treatments include over-the-counter antifungal preparations (Monistat), prescription topical agents (Terazole cream), and oral fluconazole (Diflucan). The oral treatment is more than 85% effective from a one-time dose and is much more convenient than the topical agents.

A. Oral acyclovir would be used to treat or prophylax against herpes simplex virus (HSV) lesions.

B. Topical acyclovir is more often used for herpes labialis or herpetic lesions on the upper lip than for herpes vaginalis or vulvar lesions.

C. Metronidazole can be used to treat bacterial vaginosis. Common dosing regimens include 500 mg PO BID and 250 mg PO TID.

D. Metronidazole can also be given in a vaginal preparation (Metro-gel).

64. | **C.** Rh incompatibility is a serious problem that can present in pregnancy. It occurs in the setting of an Rh-negative mother and an Rh-positive fetus. At some point during the pregnancy, but particularly at delivery, a feto-maternal hemorrhage typically occurs that leads to maternal production of IgG antibodies to Rh-positive erythrocytes. Because these antibodies can freely cross the placenta, they attack fetal blood, leading to a hemolytic anemia and erythroblastosis fetalis. The first child is usually safer from this fate than subsequent children, because blood mixing does not occur until late in pregnancy or at birth, which does not allow enough time for maternal generation of antibodies to affect the fetus. Prevention of Rh sensitization is accomplished by giving all Rh-negative pregnant women IM injections of IgG (RhoGAM) at 26 to 28 weeks of pregnancy and postpartum if the fetus is Rh-positive. Rh factor is screened for at the first prenatal visit; also at this visit, a broad antibody screen to all of the erythrocyte antigens is performed, as some of these antigens more rarely cause hemolysis in the fetus.

A. The triple screen is calibrated to screen between 15 and 20 weeks of gestation.

B. Screening for gestational diabetes is usually done at 26 to 28 weeks GA, as it is dependent upon the increasing production of the human chorionic somatomammotropin by the placenta.

D. GBS culture is usually performed at 36 weeks of gestation.

E. Pelvic US is typically not performed until 18 to 20 weeks GA, unless it is required for dating in the setting of unknown LMP.

65. **D.** Antepartum antiretroviral therapy is the central treatment modality for reducing the risk of vertical transmission in HIV-positive women. The recommended regimen consists of zidovudine (ZDV; for women with low viral loads) or a combination of zidovudine, another nucleoside analog, and either a nonnucleoside analog or a protease inhibitor (for women with viral loads exceeding 1000 or those who desire combination therapy despite low viral loads). Patients who are compliant with antiretroviral therapy decrease the risk of transmission (which is 25% if untreated) by more than 60%. Delivery by cesarean section was once recommended for all HIV-positive women, as it reduces fetal exposure to maternal HIV and has been shown to clearly reduce the risk of vertical transmission in women who have not taken antiretroviral therapy. Currently, for women who have received appropriate antiretroviral therapy and achieve undetectable viral loads, cesarean delivery is thought to be of very marginal value, if any, and is usually reserved for obstetrical indications.

A. Treatment should be initiated regardless of viral load, as vertical transmission is possible even when viral mRNA is undetectable.

B. Intrapartum ZDV and short courses of antepartum ZDV (e.g., beginning at 36 weeks) have been shown to reduce transmission rates, but these strategies are not as effective as prolonged combination therapy. These short-course antepartum regimens play an important role in countries where antiretroviral medications are prohibitively expensive, but they are not the standard of care in the United States. Although the majority of vertical transmission is believed to be intrapartum, the virus is also passed transplacentally, and any intervention limited to the perinatal period will not address this additional risk.

C. Some concerns have been raised about the effects of antiretroviral medications on the fetus, but these are thought to be outweighed by the risk of transmitting the virus if they are withheld. In general, optimal therapy should not be altered because a patient is pregnant. For patients who are known to be HIV infected before pregnancy, some controversy exists regarding whether these drugs can be held during the critical period for organogenesis. Depending on the clinical situation, treatment may be delayed until 12 weeks gestation. At 17 weeks GA, this patient should clearly begin therapy.

E. Invasive monitoring is a risk factor for vertical transmission and should be avoided whenever possible. Other peripartum risk factors for increased rates of transmission include prolonged rupture of membranes and genital ulceration.

66. **B.** Vertical transmission of HIV occurs not only transplacentally and during birth, but also via breast milk. In the United States, where alternative sources of infant nutrition are readily available, breastfeeding by HIV-positive mothers is absolutely contraindicated. The patient needs to be made aware of the risk that breastfeeding poses to her newborn. In developing countries, where alternative infant nutrition is often not available, most infants are breastfed, which leads to high rates of vertical transmission.

A. HIV is known to be expressed in breast milk, and breastfeeding carries an increased risk of transmitting the virus.

C. Breast milk offers multiple advantages for the neonate over formula feeding, including provision of passive immunity, but the risk of transmitting the virus clearly outweighs these benefits.

D. A protective effect of maternal immunoglobulins has not been demonstrated, and the risk of transmitting the virus outweighs any theoretical benefit.

E. While several antiretroviral drugs (e.g., ZDV, 3TC, and nevirapine) have been shown to be present in breast milk, a protective effect has not been demonstrated, and the risk of transmitting the virus outweighs any theoretical benefit. ZDV can be given directly to high-risk neonates.

67. | **B.** There is a threefold increase in congenital anomalies in patients with overt (pregestational) diabetes, but this increase is not seen in true gestational diabetes. This patient's elevated 3-hour OGTT could, of course, represent the unmasking of pregestational diabetes, but this patient has no pertinent positive features in her history. Statistically, the majority of diabetes diagnosed for the first time in pregnancy is true pregnancy-induced diabetes, depending on the patient population and their prepregnancy risk.

A. Pregestational maternal diabetes is clearly associated with an increase in congenital anomalies. Cardiac abnormalities and neural tube defects are the most common anomalies; sacral agenesis, while less common, is an anomaly highly specific to diabetes.

C. Early sonography can detect some malformations associated with diabetes (e.g., anencephaly), but many other congenital anomalies (e.g., cardiac defects) may not be apparent until later in gestation (18 to 20 weeks).

D. Diabetes—whether gestational or overt—is not independently associated with an increased risk of chromosomal abnormalities.

E. While oral hypoglycemic agents are a recent addition to the armamentarium to treat patients with GD, they would not decrease the risk of fetal anomalies at this GA. Although some concerns had been voiced over the use of these agents, and a weak and theoretical association with fetal nephrotoxicity and hypoglycemia had been hypothesized, recent studies do not suggest that either of these outcomes is of concern. Now that this patient has been diagnosed with GD, she should be counseled regarding diet and exercise, and she should check her blood sugars four times per day. If they remain persistently elevated despite these measures, oral hypoglycemic agents or insulin can be initiated.

68. | **C.** This patient's history is a classic presentation of one of the uterine outflow obstruction syndromes. These syndromes include imperforate hymen, transverse vaginal septum, and vaginal agenesis with either a rudimentary uterine horn or entire uterus. When these patients go through menarche, the lack of vaginal egress of menses leads to retrograde menstrual flow into the peritoneal cavity and subsequent cyclic pain. In addition, patients with imperforate hymen and transverse vaginal septum can experience a buildup of menses that collects in the upper vagina; this buildup can stretch over time and contain a large volume of old menstrual discharge. In this case, the diagnosis is either imperforate hymen or transverse vaginal septum because of the fullness noted by the patient and the clinician. The latter is the more likely diagnosis because a normal, patent hymenal ring is noted.

A. Testicular feminization also may present with a foreshortened vagina. Because affected patients do not have a uterus, however, the history regarding cyclical pain is inconsistent with testicular feminization.

B. Imperforate hymen is the second most likely diagnosis; it is often indistinguishable from transverse vaginal septum. However, the presence of a clear hymenal ring near the introitus with the vagina beyond confirms the diagnosis of transverse vaginal septum.

D. Labial fusion is seen more commonly in newborns, young children, or postmenopausal women secondary to a hypoestrogenic state and/or excessive androgenic state.

E. Patients with transverse vaginal septum are most likely to have a normal uterus, tubes, and ovaries.

69. **B.** 11β-Hydroxylase deficiency is found in one form of congenital adrenal hyperplasia (CAH). This enzyme catalyzes the conversion of 11-deoxycorticosterone to 11-deoxycortisol (compound S), which is one step involved in the production of cortisol. Due to the redundant pathways in which cortisol is made, cortisol deficiency is not generally observed. Buildup of the 11-deoxycorticosterone precursor due to enzyme deficiency, however, does lead to excess androgen production via shunt pathways. Hallmarks of this form of CAH include mild hirsutism, mild hypertension, and virilization.

A. 21-Hydroxylase is another enzyme involved in cortisol and aldosterone synthesis. Deficiency of this enzyme is the most common form of CAH, affecting approximately 2% of the population. Buildup of progesterone and 17α-hydroxyprogesterone due to this enzyme deficiency leads to excess production of DHEA, which is a precursor protein for androstenedione and testosterone synthesis. Virilization tends to be more severe in this disorder than in 11β-hydroxylase deficiency.

C. Aromatase converts androgens to estrogens in adipose tissue, muscle, and hepatocytes. While a deficiency in this enzyme could theoretically lead to virilization, it would not cause the large elevation in 11-deoxycorticosterone levels observed in this patient.

D. 3β-Hydroxysteroid dehydrogenase is another enzyme implicated in some forms of CAH. A deficiency of this enzyme would lead to increased levels of 17-hydroxypregnenolone. 11-Deoxycorticosterone levels would not be markedly elevated.

E. 5α-Reductase converts testosterone to dihydrotestosterone (DHT) in peripheral sites such as hair follicles. DHT is a more potent form of testosterone involved in hair growth and, during embryonic development, in the formation of various external genital structures. A deficiency in 5α-reductase would not affect 11-deoxycorticosterone levels.

70. **E.** The characteristics on physical exam are more consistent with a benign mass, but any adnexal mass in a postmenopausal woman is considered cancer until proven otherwise. While the large majority of women of reproductive age with this presentation will be found to have functional cysts or other benign processes, an ovarian mass in a woman older than age 50 is more likely to be malignant than benign. If this patient were younger and premenopausal, the chances of malignancy would be sufficiently small that (after appropriate imaging) she could be simply observed for probable resolution of the mass (with no further action required at this time). In contrast, a postmenopausal patient with a mass larger than 3 cm should be scheduled for exploratory surgery.

A. Although malignant tumors are more commonly unilateral than bilateral, the finding of a bilateral mass carries a greater risk of malignancy than does the finding a unilateral mass.

B. A fixed mass is suggestive of malignancy.

C. An irregular mass is suggestive of malignancy.

D. A nodular cul-de-sac is suggestive of malignancy that has spread to the pelvic cavity.

71. **D.** A septated mass is concerning for malignancy.

A. A solid mass is more suggestive of malignancy.

B. Masses larger than 5 cm are more likely to be malignant than are smaller masses.

C. Irregular contours are suggestive of malignancy.

E. Ascites are suggestive of malignancy.

72. **C.** Many of the major risk factors for ovarian cancer, other than family history, are thought to be secondary to an increased period of "chronic uninterrupted ovulation." Nulliparity is a very strong risk factor, as it contributes to this effect. Similar risk factors include early menarche and late menopause.

A. The average age of menopause in the United States is 50 to 51 years, so this patient's menopause would not be considered late onset.

B. OCPs have been found to be significantly protective against ovarian cancer, presumably through suppression of ovulation. Five years' use of OCPs has been shown to reduce the risk of ovarian cancer in a nulliparous woman by about half.

D. Tubal ligation is associated with a decreased risk of ovarian cancer. One hypothesis is that disruption of communication between the ovary and the external environment may limit exposure to carcinogens ascending the reproductive tract.

E. Infertility treatment, including clomiphene citrate, has not been shown to be an independent risk factor for ovarian cancer. Infertility itself is a risk factor (presumably ovarian dysfunction leads to both infertility and a greater risk of malignancy), and as a result there is a noncausal association between women who have received infertility treatment and the risk of ovarian cancer. This patient is presumably not infertile (with the diagnosis of male factor) and does not have this increased risk.

73. **B.** The history is consistent with development of a breast abscess in the setting of mastitis. Approximately 10% of women with mastitis develop a breast abscess despite antibiosis. The next appropriate step in evaluation is to get a breast US not only to confirm a breast abscess but also to evaluate the location and extent of the abscess. Abscesses that undermine the nipple may jeopardize the vascular supply of the nipple and require consultation with the general or plastic surgery service.

A. Despite the patient's concerning family history, her clinical course is more consistent with an abscess than breast cancer. Core biopsies are done in evaluation of solid breast masses that are concerning for a neoplasm.

C. In this patient with a difficult exam, it is not entirely clear whether she has an abscess. However, if there is an abscess on US, the patient will subsequently need incision and drainage of the abscess. Cultures and sensitivity of the purulent fluid from the abscess should be sent because many babies (and thus organisms of mastitis and subsequent abscesses) are colonized with methicillin-resistant staphylococcal strains while in the nursery during their newborn hospitalization.

D. US is the standard imaging for breast abscesses; a CT scan is not warranted.

E. Given the progressive nature of the breast process and outpatient-regimen failure, reevaluation in 1 week would be inappropriate.

74. **A.** *Staphylococcus aureus* is the most common pathogen in mastitis and breast abscesses. The organism usually arises from the infant's mouth and nose and enters via a crack or fissure in the nipple. Thus, it is safe, and recommended, that the mother continue to feed her infant from the infected breast. Good breast care and routine use of emollient creams, such as lanolin, help prevent nipple fissures. Proper breast care should be a routine part of postpartum teaching.

B. *Staphylococcus epidermidis* is part of normal skin flora, but is not a common cause of mastitis.

C. *Pseudomonas* is a more common pathogen of the respiratory or urinary tract.

D. *Propionobacterium acnes* is the bacteria most commonly associated with acne.

E. *Lactococcal ductalis* is not a real organism.

75. **C.** This woman's symptoms are most consistent with postpartum blues, which typically has an onset on postpartum days 2–6 and subsides by 2 weeks after parturition. Postpartum blues occur in approximately 50% of new mothers.

A. Postpartum depression occurs in approximately 10% of new mothers and usually has an onset at 3 to 6 months after delivery. Postpartum depression is diagnosed by the presence of at least five of the following symptoms that have at least a 2-week duration: depressed mood most of the day, diminished pleasure and interest in activities, weight changes without intentional effort to cause such, insomnia or hypersomnia, psychomotor agitation or retardation, fatigue, feelings of worthlessness or excessive guilt, difficulty concentrating or recurrent thoughts of death or suicide without a specific plan or attempt.

B. Bipolar disorder is characterized by alternating periods of depression and mania. The short nature of this patient's mood swings are inconsistent with bipolar disorder. Bipolar disorder cannot be diagnosed based on 4 days of behavior.

D. Malingering is the intentional faking of physical or psychological illness or symptoms to gain something—often medication, disability, or money. Neither the patient nor her husband are malingering, nor is there evidence that any of the reported symptoms are not legitimate.

E. Postpartum psychosis is rare. Women who have an underlying depressive, manic, schizophrenic, or schizoaffective disorder, or who have a history of a severe life event in the prior year are predisposed to its development.

76. | **B.** Approximately one fourth of women who have had a postpartum mental disorder will suffer from a recurrent event with a future pregnancy. Therefore, patients with prior episodes of postpartum depression should have a number of prophylactic measures taken, including an intact support environment of family and friends, appointments with professional counseling postpartum, and antidepressant medications.

A, C, D, E. All of these are incorrect.

77. | **C.** A Pap smear is a screening test and does not give a pathological tissue diagnosis. According to the Bethesda System, the appropriate next step in evaluation after a Pap smear is reported as HSIL is to perform a colposcopy and ECC with biopsies as indicated.

A. A CKC is a treatment procedure that is done only after a tissue diagnosis is obtained. Although they were very popular in the past, cold knife cones have since been largely replaced by LEEPs. The advantage of a CKC over an LEEP is easier evaluation of the tissue borders by the pathologist. If the patient's colposcopy evaluation reveals a high-grade lesion, conization would be indicated at that point.

B. This is one standard-of-care option (the other being to go directly to colposcopy and ECC) for LSIL, but not for HSIL.

D. Cryotherapy is a treatment procedure once a tissue diagnosis is obtained. To be a candidate for cryotherapy, a patient must have had a "satisfactory" colposcopy (the entire TZ was visualized) and show no evidence of advanced disease.

E. Bacterial vaginosis does not lead to HSIL. Thus, it would not be appropriate to retreat the patient and then to repeat the Pap smear. Vaginal infections such as *Gardnerella* vaginitis, chlamydia, candidiasis, gonorrhea, and trichomoniasis can lead to a Pap smear being read as "reactive" or "inflammatory." With either of these Pap smear reports, it would be appropriate to treat the infection and repeat the Pap smear.

78. **B.** Antepartum testing that is performed beyond 41 or 42 weeks GA in pregnancy is called post-dates testing. The nonstress test shown has two fetal heart rate accelerations that are at least 15 beats per minute higher than the baseline and is deemed reactive and thus reassuring. Patients with reassuring testing have been shown to have lower rates of IUFD as compared to high-risk patients without testing. Options for testing include the following: nonstress test (NST), contraction stress test (CST), modified biophysical profile (BPP, consisting of an NST and amniotic fluid assessment), and a complete BPP (evaluation of five diagnostic criteria including fetal tone, movement, and breathing motion, along with amniotic fluid assessment and an NST). In many high-risk pregnancies, this testing is begun between 32 and 34 weeks of gestation.

A. GD is diagnosed early in the third trimester (if not earlier). It is never tested for in the post-dates period.

C. The likelihood of meconium in the amniotic fluid increases with GA. Its most dangerous complication is the risk of meconium aspiration syndrome, which carries a high rate of morbidity for the fetus. This syndrome cannot be identified by a nonstress test.

D. Macrosomia (fetal weight greater than 4000 to 4500 g by varying definitions) is seen at higher rates in post-dates pregnancies. It is also associated with increased rates of cesarean delivery and shoulder dystocia at birth. This condition cannot be identified by a nonstress test.

E. Patients with preeclampsia should undergo early antepartum testing starting at 32 to 34 weeks GA. There is no association between an abnormal nonstress test and development of preeclampsia.

79. **D.** There is a strong association between cervical dysplasia and cervical cancer with HPV. In particular, the subtypes that put one at risk include 16, 18, and 31; in contrast, subtypes 6 and 11 predispose to condyloma formation.

A. The average length of time to the development of cervical cancer with CIN I is 7 to 10 years, whereas CIN II can develop into carcinoma in 3 to 4 years. However, some lesions progress much faster, so most patients are managed aggressively.

B. Approximately 60% of CIN I lesions resolve spontaneously.

C, E. The next step in the management of a CIN I lesion would be scheduled colposcopy and directed biopsy. Colposcopy allows a better view of the cervix and uses acetic acid to bring out the possible lesions by turning them white. Once a formal diagnosis is made, CIN I lesions are usually followed every 3 to 6 months with colposcopy until the lesions either regress or progress. If a diagnosis is made at that time, cryotherapy or laser can be used. However, an excisional procedure that can demonstrate clear margins is often the procedure of choice with either LEEP or a CKC biopsy.

80. **D.** Vulvar carcinoma accounts for 4% of gynecologic malignancies, with 90% of cases involving the squamous cell variety. It typically arises in postmenopausal women 65 to 70 years of age, and the most common presenting complaint is vulvar pruritis. Lesions most commonly arise in the inferior two-thirds of either labium majus. A punch biopsy should be performed.

A. Topical estrogen is often prescribed to relieve symptoms of postmenopausal vaginal atrophy. However, the presence of an ulcer is not consistent with routine atrophy.

B. Topical steroids are used to treat lichen sclerosus, lichen simplex chronicus, psoriasis, and lichen planus. The described lesion is not typical for any of these diagnoses, and delay of further evaluation would be inappropriate.

C. One needs a tissue diagnosis prior to performing a therapeutic excisional procedure, and wide local vulvar excisions are not done in the office.

E. Atrophy with pruritis is quite common in postmenopausal women and prescription of HRT can alleviate these symptoms in appropriate patients. However, this patient has a discrete ulcerated lesion that is suspicious for vulvar carcinoma and should be biopsied.

81. **B.** The upper vagina is the most common place for vaginal carcinoma to arise. The most common complaint with vaginal cancer is a vaginal discharge that is often bloody. However, urinary symptoms can arise with bulky disease given the close proximity of the upper vagina to the bladder neck.

A, C, D. These are not the most common locations for vaginal carcinoma to arise. The labia majora are not part of the vagina.

E. Vaginal cancer has a predilection for the upper vagina.

82. **C.** The upper vagina is drained by the internal and common iliac nodes.

A. Vaginal cancer does not spread hematogenously.

B. The lower vagina is drained by the regional nodes in the femoral triangle.

D. The supraclavicular nodes are not in the immediate chain of nodes that drain the genitourinary system. The presence of a palpable supraclavicular node should alert the clinician to the possibility of other malignancies—specifically, lung, breast, GI, and hematogenous.

E. The posterior cervical chain of nodes is in the neck, not the pelvis. These nodes are commonly enlarged with viral and oropharyngeal infections (strep pharyngitis).

83. **C.** Stage III extends to the pelvic sidewall. Stage IV extends beyond the true pelvis or involves the mucosa of the bladder or rectum. This patient has at least Stage III disease but may well have Stage IV disease. Her urinary symptoms could be secondary either to mucosal invasion or mass compression. Five-year survival rates are 40% for Stage III disease and 0% for Stage IV disease.

A. Stage I is limited to the vaginal mucosa.

B. Stage II involves the submucosa but does not extend to the sidewall.

D. There is no Stage V.

E. Vaginal cancer is clinically staged, not pathologically staged.

84. | **C.** Induction of labor has been associated with a two- to fivefold increase in the rate of uterine rupture. This rate of uterine rupture is further increased by the use of prostaglandins for induction by three- to fourfold. Thus, in most patients undergoing indicated induction of labor who had a prior cesarean delivery, mechanical means with a Foley bulb are typically utilized.

A. The risk of uterine rupture in women with one prior low transverse cesarean scar is 0.5% to 1%. This risk would be increased if the patient underwent induction of labor, but would still be below the 5% to 10% range.

B. Management of uterine rupture requires immediate laparotomy, delivery of the fetus, and repair of the rupture site or hysterectomy if bleeding cannot be controlled.

D. In some early studies, fetal mortality in the event of uterine rupture was as high as 30% to 40%. However, with the ready availability of obstetricians and anesthesiologists, as well as earlier recognition of uterine rupture, mortality rates in one recent large study were closer to 5%.

E. Injudicious use of oxytocin during labor increases the risk of uterine rupture in patients with prior uterine scars.

85. | **B.** Post-term pregnancies are at increased risk for fetal demise, macrosomia, meconium aspiration, and oligohydramnios. The management of post-term pregnancy includes more frequent office visits, increased fetal testing, and plans for eventual labor induction. This patient has a favorable cervix for induction. Beyond 42 weeks, however, most patients will be counseled toward labor induction regardless of the cervical exam.

A. The opposite is true, with amniotic fluid volume decreasing toward the end of pregnancy.

C. The risk of Rh sensitization does not increase with postdates pregnancy.

D. The opposite is true, with the rate of macrosomia increasing among post-term pregnancies. The risk of low birthweight (less than 2500 g) would be quite low among post-term infants.

E. The rate of respiratory distress syndrome falls with increasing GA until 39 weeks, at which point it remains stable.

86. | **A.** Twin–twin transfusion syndrome can occur in monochorionic/diamnionic twin gestations. Vascular communication between twins can result in one fetus with hypervolemia, cardiomegaly, glomerulotubal hypertrophy, edema, ascites, and polyhydramnios, while the other twin has hypovolemia, growth restriction, and oligohydramnios. The US image shows fetal ascites and large pleural effusions.

B. Rh sensitization may occur when an Rh-negative woman is exposed to fetal blood that is Rh-positive, resulting in maternal production of antibodies (i.e., sensitization). In sensitized patients with Rh-positive fetuses, these antibodies can cross the placenta and cause hemolysis of fetal blood cells, leading to varying degrees of fetal anemia and possibly erythroblastosis fetalis.

C. In "Siamese" twinning, or conjoined twinning, the fetuses are monochorionic/monoamniotic (i.e., they share one placenta and an amniotic sac).

D. This is not a normal variant of twinning.

E. Congenital rubella syndrome, like any teratogenic infection, would be likely to affect both twins.

87. **C. In reproductive-age women, pregnancy is the most common cause of secondary amenorrhea. In this patient who has a history of being sexually active, a urine pregnancy test should be performed in the office to obtain a diagnosis. The other clue in her history is the weight gain despite her athletic training.**

A. Kallmann's syndrome involves a congenital absence of GnRH (commonly associated with anosmia) and is a hypothalamic cause of primary amenorrhea. Primary amenorrhea is the absence of menses in women who have not undergone menarche by age 16 or who have not begun menstruating by 4 years after thelarche.

B. Secondary amenorrhea is the absence of menses for three menstrual cycles or a total of 6 months in a woman who has had previously normal menses. Common causes of secondary amenorrhea include pregnancy, anatomic abnormalities (e.g., Asherman's syndrome), ovarian dysfunction, hypothyroidism, prolactinomas and hyperprolactinemia, and CNS or hypothalamic disorders.

D, E. Exercise and stress can both lead to hypothalamic dysfunction, producing amenorrhea. Certainly in this patient who is a competitive athlete as well as likely to have a stressful academic life, these issues would be the next in line as likely etiologies for her secondary amenorrhea.

88. **D. Screening for trisomy 18 is via serum screening, of which MSAFP is a part. Both trisomy 18 and trisomy 21 (Down syndrome) are increased with an MSAFP value that is lower than normal. The triple screen (MSAFP, estriol, and β-hcG) differ between trisomy 18 and Down syndrome in that all three values are diminished in trisomy 18, whereas β-hcG is actually increased in the setting of Down syndrome.**

A. In cases of anencephaly, AFP is released from the neural tissue into the amniotic fluid, and subsequently crosses into maternal circulation leading to higher MSAFP levels.

B. Because of the increased number of fetuses, more AFP crosses into the maternal circulation.

C. AFP is primarily produced in the fetal neural tissue and liver. Thus any break in the fetal abdominal integument can allow increased levels to be released into the amniotic fluid and subsequently into the maternal circulation.

E. Use of MSAFP as a screening test is dependent upon accurate dating of the pregnancy. Because MSAFP increases during the second trimester, elevated values can occur if a patient is actually several weeks further along in pregnancy than indicated by her dating.

89. **C.** Premature labor, second trimester abortions, and fetal malpresentation (i.e., breech or transverse lie) are likely due to the size limitations of a bicornuate uterus.

A. Endometriosis is not associated with a bicornuate uterus. It has been found in association with blind uterine horns.

B. In the case of uterine anomalies associated with DES use by a patient's mother, there is an increase in vaginal cancer. However, increased rates of uterine cancer have not been documented.

D. While uterine anomalies are associated with urinary tract anomalies, they are not particularly associated with increased rates of UTIs. Embryologically, the superior vagina, cervix, uterus, and fallopian tubes all originate from fusion of the paramesonephric (müllerian) ducts. The urinary tract develops from the neighboring urogenital sinus. If the paramesonephric ducts fail to fuse during embryogenesis, urinary tract anomalies can also result given the proximity of these two developing areas. Further investigation is warranted, often in the form of an intravenous pyelogram.

E. There does not appear to be a genetic component to uterine anomalies, and they are not commonly found in familial case series. Similarly, no other fetal anomalies are associated with uterine anomalies.

90. **A.** Surgery is the correct treatment for a correctable uterine anomaly including septate uterus. After successful surgical intervention, 70% to 80% of patients successfully deliver a viable fetus. A simple uterine septum can be excised hysteroscopically. Metroplasty procedures, in which a segment of the uterine wall is resected, have been utilized in cases of thicker uterine septums.

B. If one or both partners have a genetic anomaly such as a balanced translocation, Clomid and intrauterine insemination will not increase their likelihood of having a normal pregnancy. In addition to genetic counseling, this couple might consider using a donor egg or sperm.

C. Antiphospholipid antibody syndrome is typically treated with low-dose aspirin (81 mg) with or without low-dose heparin (5000 to 10,000 units SQ q12 hours). Corticosteroids have been described as an alternative treatment, but benefits from this treatment have not been supported in clinical trials.

D. Patients with recurrent pregnancy loss (RPL) and hyperprolactinemia receive bromocriptine therapy.

E. Group B *Streptococcus* is not known to cause recurrent pregnancy loss.

91. **C.** Several criteria must be met for a safe attempt at a VBAC. An obstetrician must be immediately available 24 hours a day, and an anesthesiologist must be on call. A prior classical hysterotomy (a vertical incision that extends to the fundus of the uterus) is a contraindication to TOL after prior cesarean section. Knowledge of the previous incision and no history of extension into the cervix or active portion of the uterus are also usually regarded as requirements for TOL to be allowed. In addition, patients must have signed an informed consent form for a TOL to be attempted.

A. A number of obstetric history risk factors lead to an increased risk for uterine rupture—namely, interpregnancy interval of less than 18 months, infection at the time of a prior cesarean section, single-layer closure of the prior cesarean section, and more than one prior cesarean section. While all of these increased risks should be mentioned in the counseling, none of them is considered an absolute contraindication to a subsequent trial of labor after cesarean.

B. The specific reason for previous cesarean section does not affect the safety of the cesarean delivery but affects the likelihood of successful VBAC.

D. Kerr and Kronig incisions are both associated with a low rate of uterine rupture during a subsequent trial of labor (0.5% to 1%). Classical cesarean section, which extends above the insertion of the round ligaments, has been associated with a 6% to 12% rate of uterine rupture and is a contraindication to TOL.

E. A postpartum hemorrhage after VBAC does not affect a safe attempt at vaginal delivery. At the same time, preparations must be made to ensure that morbidity is limited if the patient were to experience a repeat hemorrhage (e.g., confirm availability of blood products).

92. **C.** An Rh-negative mother who is sensitized against anti-D creates IgG antibodies that cross the placenta and can attack fetal erythrocytes, leading to fetal hemolytic anemia and eventually high output failure, known as fetal hydrops. In this case, the father is known to be Rh-positive because he previously fathered an Rh-positive child with an Rh-negative woman; he is heterozygous because he also fathered an Rh-negative child. Given the Hardy-Weinberg equation $(p^2 + 2pq + q^2 = 1$, where p = probability of dominant allele and q = probability of recessive allele), we can calculate several probabilities. The numerator is half of the probability of the heterozygotes ($1/2 * 2pq = pq$). The denominator is equal to the probability of having at least one D allele ($2pq$). Thus the overall probability is $pq/(2pq) = 1/2$. It can also be seen that because the father is heterozygous, there is a 50% chance that he will pass on the D allele and a 50% chance that he will pass on the "–" allele. In this case, "–" is used instead of "d" because there is no recessive allele.

A. With no other information, there is a $2pq$ probability of being heterozygous. This equals $2 \times 0.4 \times 0.6 = 0.48$ in Caucasians. However, this patient's husband previously fathered an Rh-negative child and an Rh-positive child, so he must be heterozygous.

B. The husband is Rh-positive.

D. RhoGAM has no use in patients who are already sensitized.

E. As long as the antibody titer remains at 1:8 or lower, there is no reason to perform any amniocenteses. Serial amniocenteses for hemoglobin breakdown products are only necessary at titers of 1:16 or beyond.

93. C. Bleeding in a postmenopausal woman is assumed to be endometrial cancer until proven otherwise. This patient also has several risk factors for endometrial hyperplasia or carcinoma—namely, obesity, nulliparity, late menopause (more than 55 years old at menopause), and likely chronic anovulation given her history of irregular menses. The most important evaluation of bleeding in a postmenopausal woman is an office endometrial biopsy (EMB). Bleeding is suspicious for endometrial hyperplasia or carcinoma, and a tissue sample is necessary for a pathologic diagnosis. Hyperplasia is the proliferation or overgrowth of the glands and stroma of the endometrium. It can result in histologic changes (simple or complex) of the cellular architecture with or without cellular atypia. There is a spectrum of hyperplasia ranging from simple hyperplasia without atypia (fairly benign) to atypical complex hyperplasia that progresses to carcinoma in approximately 29% of untreated cases.

A. US can offer some reassurance if the endometrial strip is smaller than 5 mm and homogeneous. However, a tissue diagnosis is still warranted.

B. Although patient reassurance is always an important part of patient care, investigating the source of her bleeding is most important.

D. A Pap smear is helpful in screening for cervical cancer.

E. If the patient is unable to tolerate an office EMB, a D&C would be the next best means of evaluation.

94. C. This patient's lesion is caused by chronic irritation of the vulva by her routine pad use leading to a hypertrophic area, called lichen simplex chronicus. It most likely started as a moist, erythematous lesion and, with continued abrasion from the pads and the patient's scratching, transformed into a white raised lesion. The best treatment is hydrocortisone cream.

A. Contact dermatitis can be caused by an irritant in the pads that the patient uses for her incontinence, but the time course is inconsistent, typically lasting hours rather than weeks. The most common cause of contact dermatitis is oleoresin found in poison ivy and oak.

B. Vaginitis due to yeast infection is a common diagnosis. Affected patients complain of vaginal pruritis, burning, and vaginal discharge. Exam reveals vulvar edema and a discharge that exhibits hyphae and spores on microscopic evaluation.

D. Lichen sclerosus et atrophicus is a similar condition often diagnosed in postmenopausal women secondary to atrophy due to decreased estrogenization of the vulvar tissue. It can also present with pruritis and white lesions, but usually involves tissue thinning. The treatment for lichen sclerosus et atrophicus is hydrocortisone cream to decrease pruritis and inflammation and 2% testosterone cream to support the atrophic epithelium.

E. A biopsy of any suspicious vulvar lesion should be examined by a pathologist because the above two conditions can easily be mistaken for vulvar cancer.

95. **A.** Choroid plexus cysts (CPCs) have been associated with trisomy 18. CPCs can be formally diagnosed by amniocentesis. Trisomy 18 can be screened for by obstetric US, which can identify the following associated major structural defects: rocker-bottom feet, clubfoot, overriding digits, omphalocele, and cerebral malformations such as holoprosencephaly.

B. The lack of a fetal skull on US exam is usually how anencephaly is diagnosed. The most severe form of neural tube defect, it is not compatible with life.

C. NTDs can be difficult to diagnose by US, but cerebral findings such as the "lemon" sign (indentation of the frontal bones) and the "banana" sign (obliteration of the posterior fossa by the cerebellar hemispheres that appear to be pulled posteriorly) can help. Most NTDs are found by elevated MSAFP on second trimester serum screening.

D. CPCs have not been associated with any long-term poor outcomes in fetuses with normal chromosomes.

E. Turner's syndrome is a sex chromosomal abnormality (45,XO) that results in a syndrome of short stature, webbed neck, shield-shaped chest, wide-spaced nipples, and often infertility. Affected women have relatively normal intelligence. Turner's syndrome has not been associated with CPCs.

96. **E.** This patient's syndrome of hirsutism and anovulation along with physical findings of acanthosis nigricans (velvety, thickened skin in the axilla and nape of the neck) is consistent with PCOS. Also known as PCOD or simply PCO, this syndromic condition was first described by Stein and Leventhal in the setting of hirsutism, virilism, anovulation, amenorrhea, and obesity. It is also associated with insulin resistance and hence type 2 diabetes. Without any other etiology for her symptoms, this diagnosis can be made. An LH:FSH ratio of greater than 3 is also used to confirm this diagnosis of exclusion, but sole reliance on this ratio can miss the diagnosis in morbidly obese anovulatory patients who have suppression of their gonadotropins and thus will not have an elevated ratio.

A, D. Ovarian tumors that can lead to hirsutism and virilism include the sex-cord mesenchymal tumors, granulosa-theca cell tumors, germ cell tumors, and the Sertoli-Leydig cell tumors. These tumors can all secrete testosterone; hence a testosterone elevation is often observed. Furthermore, virilism due to ovarian tumors usually presents more acutely with rapid onset of symptoms.

B. CAH results from a constellation of enzyme deficiencies, with the most common being an absence of 21-α-hydroxylase, which results in excess 17-α-hydroxyprogesterone and can lead to the complete inability to synthesize cortisol or mineralocorticoids. Adult-onset CAH can be quite mild, characterized by anovulation and androgenization, but should still be notable for elevated dehydroepiandrosterone sulfate (DHEA-S) and/or testosterone.

C. Testicular feminization is most commonly related to absence or dysfunction of the testosterone receptor. These patients are genetically 46,XY but are phenotypically female. Because of the testosterone receptor dysfunction, they cannot become hirsute or virilized.

97. **C.** Kegel exercises entail isometric contraction of the pubococcygeus muscles to increase their strength. Performance of regular Kegel exercises may reduce the patient's symptoms. While not always effective, Kegel exercises are noninvasive and inexpensive, and they should be used as the initial management of mild pelvic prolapse.

A. Estrogen therapy may improve mild pelvic relaxation and should be offered if the patient's symptoms do not improve with Kegel exercises.

B. Anterior repair, or anterior colporrhaphy, is surgical treatment and should be reserved for patients with severe symptoms, after conservative measures have failed.

D. Colpocleisis involves the surgical closure of the vagina and is not indicated. The procedure is usually reserved for elderly, non-sexually active women with symptomatic vaginal prolapse, who have failed to respond to other measures.

E. A pessary is a device, often made of rubber or Lucite, that is placed into the vagina to hold pelvic organs in place. It is usually used only as an alternative to surgery.

98. **A.** This patient's history and physical exam are most consistent with stress incontinence, although a formal diagnosis is usually made with urodynamics testing. The fact that she leaks only with valsalva and physical activity is consistent with stress incontinence. Her risk factors include mild pelvic relaxation, childbirth, and the postmenopausal anestrogenic state. Her positive Q-tip test on physical exam further confirms the diagnosis. Stress incontinence can be treated medically with exercises, estrogen administration, and surgical restoration of the bladder neck to its original anatomic position.

B. Urge incontinence patients feel the urge to micturate and then urine begins to leak before they can get to the bathroom.

C. Detrusor instability is one etiology of urge incontinence. In addition, patients will occasionally have detrusor instability along with stress incontinence symptoms. Various stressors such as coughing can trigger detrusor contraction, leading to an appearance of stress incontinence that is actually detrusor instability. This can be diagnosed with urodynamics that reveal a detrusor contraction several seconds after a valsalva and leakage that occurs with the detrusor contraction rather than with the valsalva.

D. Total incontinence is rare and results from complete inability to maintain continence. It is most commonly seen in patients with fistulae from the bladder to the vagina or skin, or from the urethra or ureters to the vagina.

E. Overflow incontinence results from detrusor insufficiency or areflexia; that is, the bladder wall contracts weakly or not at all. In this case, urine collects in the bladder and dribbles out when the bladder capacity is exceeded.

99. **B.** This patient presents with incompetent cervix—that is, silent, painless dilation of the cervix without contractions, usually occurring in the mid- to late second trimester. Unfortunately, most diagnoses of incompetent cervix are made when it is too late to intervene to benefit the current pregnancy. Future management is to place a prophylactic cerclage between 12 and 14 weeks of gestation. In this patient with dilation that has allowed a large portion of her membranes to prolapse into the vagina as shown in the image, there are only two reasonable forms of management. The first is termination of this pregnancy with either induction of labor or D&E. The second is expectant management, which many patients will wish to attempt in the hope of achieving a viable pregnancy (24 weeks or later GA). If the patient chooses the latter option, she must be followed with serial abdominal exams, temperatures, and WBC counts. If any signs or symptoms of infection appear, the patient should be encouraged to undergo a termination of pregnancy at that point. An emergent cerclage placement in the setting of prolapsing membranes is not advised due to the increased risk of complications such as infection and ruptured membranes.

A. Bacterial vaginosis (BV) is associated with preterm delivery and can be treated with oral metronidazole. This patient does not have BV.

C. While vaginal clindamycin is another way to treat BV, it is not indicated in this patient.

D. This patient has had no contractions, making tocolysis unnecessary at this time.

E. Betamethasone and dexamethasone have been shown to decrease rates of respiratory distress syndrome in neonates when given between 24 and 34 weeks of gestation. At this GA, the fetus is previable, so it is of little use to give antenatal corticosteroids.

100. **D.** This is a classic setup for Rh incompatibility. Because the father is Rh-positive, there is a chance he passed the Rh-positive allele to the fetus, making it Rh-positive as well. Given that the mother is Rh-negative, any exposure to Rh-positive fetal blood would induce her immune system to produce antibodies, including IgG, to Rh factor. Because IgG freely crosses the placenta, production of anti-Rh IgG could produce serious consequences for the fetus, including hemolytic anemia and hyperbilirubinemia leading to kernicterus, heart failure, ascites, and many other problems collectively known as erythroblastosis fetalis. Usually the first child is relatively protected from this condition because fetal–maternal blood mixing does not occur until late in pregnancy or at birth, and the mother does not have sufficient time to mount a strong antibody response before the baby is born. However, if this response is mounted, all future Rh-positive fetuses will be in danger of being attacked by the mother's now primed immune system. Therefore, RhoGAM (anti-Rh immunoglobulin) is given to the mother during the third trimester—even during the first pregnancy—as a precaution. These antibodies bind to the Rh-positive cells before the mother can detect them, thereby preventing an immune response from being mounted and keeping this and all future pregnancies safe from attack.

A. Amniocentesis is not indicated for an Rh-incompatibility workup. To the contrary, amniocentesis is not advisable in this patient as this procedure can lead to fetal–maternal blood mixing and subsequent sensitization, the very consequence you are trying to prevent. If amniocentesis must be performed in an Rh-negative woman, RhoGAM should be administered after the procedure.

B. See the explanation for D. Because mixing of fetal–maternal blood does not typically occur until late in pregnancy, it is entirely possible that the patient has not yet been exposed to fetal blood, and therefore has not yet mounted an immune response. There is no reason to recheck the father's Rh status.

C. Because this is their first child, it is highly unlikely that the mother will mount a sufficient immune response to cause any lasting problems in the fetus.

E. See the explanation for D. RhoGAM is certainly indicated.

Questions

Setting 3: Inpatient Facilities

You have general admitting privileges to the hospital. You may see patients in the critical care unit, the pediatrics unit, the maternity unit, or recovery room. You may also be called to see patients in the psychiatric unit. A short-stay unit serves patients who are undergoing same-day operations or who are being held for observation. There are adjacent nursing home/extended-care facilities and a detoxification unit where you may see patients.

101. A 29-year-old G$_2$P$_1$ woman at 39 2/7 weeks GA presents in active labor. She has been contracting for 4 hours and on admission is contracting painfully every 2 to 3 minutes. Her cervix is 4 cm dilated and the fetal head is at −1 station. The patient's prior labor lasted 13 hours and culminated in a spontaneous vaginal delivery of a 9 lb 4 oz boy (4200 g) after a 60-minute second stage. By US and Leopolds, this fetus, a baby girl, is approximately 3700 g. The patient progresses slowly in labor, dilating approximately 1 cm every 1 to 2 hours during the next 12 hours. At this time, she feels the urge to push; on exam, she is fully dilated, −1 station, and left occiput transverse (LOT) position. She begins the second stage. After pushing for 2 hours, station is unchanged, and the fetal position is as shown in Figure 101. The patient requests assistance with a forceps or vacuum delivery because of exhaustion. Which of the following might be considered a contraindication for forceps delivery?

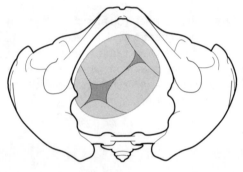

Figure 101 • Reproduced with permission from Callahan T. Blueprints Obstetrics & Gynecology. 3rd ed. Blackwell, 2004: Fig. 4-4 H, p. 34.

A. Lack of epidural anesthesia
B. Fetal station
C. Prior infant greater than 9 lb
D. Fetal position
E. Maternal exhaustion

102. A 19-year-old G$_1$P$_0$ woman at 39 5/7 GA presents with uterine contractions every 3 to 4 minutes. On exam, she is 4 cm dilated, 100% effaced, +1 station. She is admitted to labor and delivery. Over the next 2 hours, she changes her cervix to 6 cm dilation, +1 station, and left occiput anterior (LOA) position. At this point, she requests an epidural. One hour after epidural placement, her exam is unchanged at 6 cm and +1 station. Artificial rupture of the membranes (AROM, or amniotomy) is performed, and Pitocin (oxytocin) is begun for augmentation of labor. Over the ensuing 2 hours, she contracts every 3 to 5 minutes, and she changes to 7 cm and +1 station. After 2 more hours, she maintains the same exam of 7 cm and +1 station, with a position of LOA. At this point, the diagnosis of failure to progress in labor is suggested. Which of the following is most important to making this diagnosis?

A. Placement of an IUPC to measure contractions
B. Cervical change of less than 1.5 cm per hour
C. At least 2 hours of Pitocin augmentation
D. No change in station over a period of 4 hours
E. An active phase of the second stage of labor greater than 5 hours

103. A 33-year-old G_4P_3 woman at term presents in active labor at 5-cm dilation. She has a reactive fetal heart tracing with a baseline in the 150s. Contractions are occurring every 2 to 3 minutes. Estimated fetal weight is 3600 g, and she had rupture of membranes approximately 3 hours prior to presentation. During the next hour, the FHR tracing begins to show decelerations (Figure 103). These decelerations are called___ and are likely secondary to___.

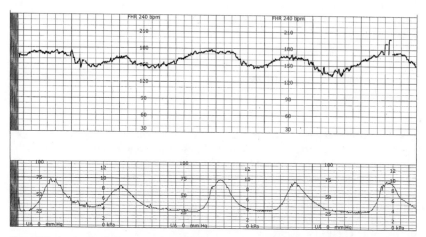

Figure 103 · Image provided by Department of Obstetrics & Gynecology, University of California, San Francisco.

A. Early decelerations; head compression
B. Variable decelerations; uteroplacental insufficiency
C. Late decelerations; uteroplacental insufficiency
D. Late decelerations; head compression
E. Early decelerations; a nuchal cord

104. A 19-year-old G_1P_0 woman at 41 2/7 weeks GA has just undergone a spontaneous vaginal delivery of a viable 4425-g boy. She had been diagnosed with preeclampsia and has been on magnesium sulfate for seizure prophylaxis for 26 hours. She spiked a fever to 101.8°F five hours ago and is being treated with cefotetan for presumed chorioamnionitis. After the delivery of the placenta, which appears intact and without obvious vessels traveling into the membranes, she begins to have a postpartum hemorrhage. During the next minute she loses 300 cc of blood, for a total of approximately 1 L. Which of the following is the most likely etiology in this clinical situation?

    A. Cervical laceration
    B. Vaginal laceration
    C. Ruptured hemorrhoidal vessels
    D. Uterine atony
    E. Retained POCs

105. A 17-year-old G_1P_0 woman at 37 2/7 weeks GA presents with blood pressures elevated to 146–158/93–102. A urine dipstick shows 2+ proteinuria. She denies headache or visual changes, but she does note some swelling of her hands. On physical exam, you note no papilledema, no right upper quadrant tenderness, brisk 3+ deep tendon reflexes (DTRs), and 2+ pitting edema of the lower extremities. She is admitted to labor and delivery, magnesium sulfate is administered to her for seizure prophylaxis, and her labor is induced. Which of the following lab tests, if the results are elevated, would help make the diagnosis of HELLP syndrome?

    A. Creatinine
    B. Hematocrit
    C. Aspartate transaminase (AST)
    D. Uric acid
    E. Platelet count

106. A 32-year-old G_2P_1 woman presents at 36 4/7 weeks GA with a dichorionic/diamnionic twin gestation. Her twin gestation was diagnosed by US at 8 weeks. An anatomic survey and amniocentesis were performed at 17 weeks, and both were normal. The fetal karyotypes are 46,XY and 46,XX. The patient had another US at 29 weeks GA, which showed concordant fetal growth with percentile weights of 46% and 57%, respectively. The patient now presents with contractions every 2 to 3 minutes and a cervical exam of 2 cm dilation, 90% effacement, and 0 station. You counsel her that which of the following is commonly accepted in the delivery of twins?

A. Trial of labor for breech-presenting twin, cephalic second twin
B. High-dose Pitocin after delivery of the first twin to remove the placenta
C. Immediate delivery of the second twin with forceps, even if the cervix is no longer fully dilated
D. Elective cesarean delivery for a cephalic-presenting first twin and cephalic-presenting second twin
E. After delivery of the first twin, immediate breech extraction of the second twin

107. A 28-year-old G_3P_2 woman at 38 2/7 weeks GA presents in active labor, 4 cm dilated, 90% effaced, and +1 station. The fetus is breech, which it had been 2 weeks earlier. A prior attempt at external cephalic version failed. CT scan for pelvimetry found the pelvis to be adequate for breech delivery. After a discussion of the risks and benefits of breech delivery with her primary obstetrician, the patient elects to attempt a trial of labor. Which of the following is generally considered necessary in the decision to allow a trial of labor for a breech-presenting fetus?

A. Estimated fetal weight less than 4500 g
B. Fetal head is flexed
C. Patient has an epidural for anesthesia
D. Prior vaginal delivery
E. No prior cesarean deliveries

108. A 22-year-old G_1P_0 woman at 29 2/7 weeks GA presents with complaints of recurrent lower back pain. She is placed on the fetal heart monitor and tocometer and is found to be contracting every 2 to 3 minutes. She has no complaints of fluid leakage, but notes that she had some spotting the last time she urinated. A sterile speculum exam is negative for pooling, nitrazine, and ferning. On sterile vaginal exam, she is 2 cm dilated, 85% effaced, at +1 station, and cephalic presenting. Which of the following management choices has been demonstrated to have the greatest effect on neonatal outcomes?

A. 6-g IV bolus of magnesium sulfate
B. 500-mg IV bolus of erythromycin
C. 12-mg IM dose of betamethasone
D. 0.25-mg SC dose of terbutaline
E. 5-millions unit IV dose of penicillin

109. A 31-year-old G_2P_1 patient at 37 2/7 weeks GA presents complaining of leaking clear fluid for the last hour. One hour prior to presenting, she had a large gush of about 100 cc of fluid, and has had smaller leaks since then. She has not experienced any contractions or bleeding. On sterile speculum exam, you note a small pool of clear fluid in the vagina. A sample of this fluid is dried on a slide (Figure 109). On inspection, the cervix is long and closed. The FHR tracing is reactive and without decelerations. Which of the following is the most commonly accepted approach to management based on existing literature?

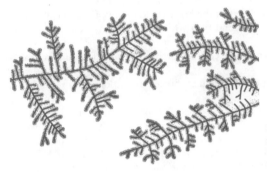

Figure 109 • Reproduced with permission from Marbas L. Blueprints Clinical Procedures. Blackwell, 2004: Fig. 60-1, p. 174.

A. Discharge home
B. Immediate induction of labor with oxytocin
C. Treat with antibiotics
D. Treat with a course of betamethasone
E. Expectant management at home for the next 96 hours

110. A 23-year-old G_1P_0 woman presents in active labor. She progresses rapidly to complete dilation and undergoes a 30-minute second stage. She delivers a viable fetus with Apgar scores of 8 and 9. Upon inspection of the fetus, you note that the infant has either an enlarged clitoris or a very small penis, and partially fused labioscrotal swellings. You order a 17-hydroxyprogesterone test, which is elevated. In addition to telling the patient and her husband the likely sex of the child, you also mention that which of the following treatments will be necessary for the child?

A. Immediate surgery to correct the genitalia
B. Estradiol
C. Progesterone
D. Testosterone
E. Prednisone

111. A 26-year-old G_1P_0 woman presents in active labor at 39 2/7 weeks GA. She had an uncomplicated antepartum course and has a history of scleroderma. Her disease is currently under control with the use of prednisone. In labor, you begin stress-dose steroids. Two hours later, you are called by nursing for a prolonged deceleration. Upon pelvic exam, you note a prolapsed umbilical cord beyond the fetal head. The FHR tracing is obtained (Figure 111). The patient is moved to the operating room (OR) for an emergent cesarean delivery as you continue to elevate the fetal head off the umbilical cord. In the OR, the obstetric anesthesiologist asks about your preference for anesthesia. What is your response?

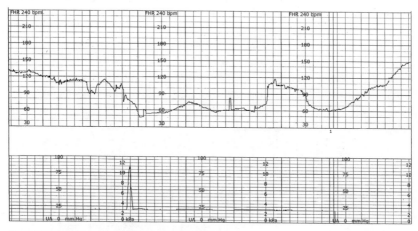

Figure 111 · Image provided by Department of Obstetrics & Gynecology, University of California, San Francisco.

A. Epidural anesthesia is preferred
B. Spinal anesthesia is preferred
C. She needs to be given general anesthesia
D. You can use local anesthesia with conscious sedation
E. A pudendal block can be placed

112. A 31-year-old G_2P_1 woman presents in active labor at 39 5/7 weeks GA. She is 5 cm dilated, 90% effaced, and +1 station. The FHR tracing is reassuring with no decelerations, and the tocometer reveals contractions every 2 to 3 minutes. The patient has had an uncomplicated prenatal course. Her obstetrical history is remarkable for a cesarean delivery 4 years ago for failure to progress past 7-cm dilation. On labor and delivery, she requests an epidural, which is placed without complication. On her next exam 2 hours later, she is 7 cm dilated and +2 station, but her contractions have decreased to every 5 to 7 minutes. She is begun on oxytocin for augmentation. An hour later, the FHR tracing appears as in Figure 112. On exam, the cervix is now 8 cm dilated, but the fetal head cannot be easily palpated, indicating that it is at least above −3 station. What is the next step in the management of this patient?

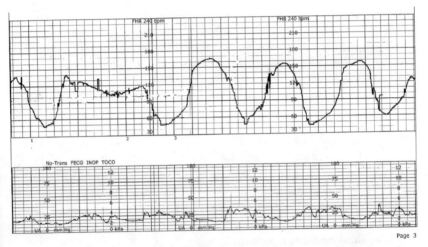

Page 3

Figure 112 • Image provided by Department of Obstetrics & Gynecology, University of California, San Francisco.

A. Fetal scalp pH
B. Cesarean delivery
C. Forceps delivery
D. Expectant management
E. Restart Pitocin to help bring the head back down

113. A 57-year-old woman underwent a total abdominal hysterectomy and bilateral salpingo-oophorectomy (TAH-BSO) with bilateral pelvic lymph node sampling for stage I, grade III endometrial cancer. She was discharged home on postoperative day 3 with oral cephalexin (Keflex) because of a wound cellulitis. She now returns 2 days later with complaints of leaking pus from the lateral edge of the incision. On physical exam she is obese, with a Pfannenstiel skin incision that has surrounding erythema 3 to 4 cm superiorly. The left aspect of the incision is slightly open; when you palpate the area, a small amount of thick, yellowish discharge is extruded. You attempt to probe the incision with a cotton swab, but it cannot be passed into the small opening. What is your next step?

A. Start the patient on IV antibiotics
B. Schedule the patient for an incision and drainage of the wound in the OR
C. Using local anesthesia, open the lateral edge of the incision with a scalpel for further exploration
D. Using an IV catheter, irrigate the small opening at the lateral edge of the incision
E. Order a CT scan to examine the incision

114. A 66-year-old woman is 12 hours postoperatively from an exploratory laparotomy and debulking procedure for ovarian cancer. At the time of the surgery, approximately 4 L of ascites was removed from the abdomen. You are called by nursing because the patient has made only 15 cc of urine over the last hour. Her fluid intake and output for the day are recorded in Table 114. Over the past 3 hours her urine output has progressively slowed from 30 cc/h to 25 cc/h and finally 15 cc/h. What is the next step in this patient's management?

■ TABLE 114	Fluid Balance	
	In	Out
Operating room	1600 cc crystalloid	700 cc EBL, 200 cc urine
Postoperative	1200 cc crystalloid	250 cc drains, 520 cc urine

A. Bolus 500 cc IV crystalloid
B. Bolus 2000 cc IV crystalloid
C. Bolus IV colloid, salt-poor albumin
D. IV furosemide (Lasix)
E. PO furosemide (Lasix)

115. A 53-year-old obese woman is undergoing a TAH-BSO for stage I, grade I endometrial cancer. During the procedure, a clamp on the left uterine artery slips and the patient loses a total of 1500 cc of blood. Her preoperative hematocrit was 42. During the procedure, she received 3500 cc of crystalloid. At the end of the procedure, there was no obvious bleeding from this pedicle. Six hours postoperatively, she has a hematocrit drawn, which returns 28. At this time, her blood pressure is 108/64 and her heart rate is 88. Her urine output over the prior 3 hours has been 55 cc, 50 cc, and 65 cc. What is the next step in this patient's management?

A. Follow serial hematocrits
B. This is an appropriate drop—check hematocrit in the morning
C. Return to operating room for immediate exploration
D. Transfuse 2 units of PRBCs
E. Check PT/PTT

116. A 23-year-old woman presents 3 days postoperatively with complaints of abdominal pain and fever. She had undergone a laparoscopic resection and fulguration of endometriosis with unipolar cautery. She is seen in the ED by her primary physician. On physical exam, she has a temperature of 101.4°F, tachycardia to the 120s, and an abdominal exam with rebound tenderness. Her bimanual exam shows some slight cervical motion tenderness. She is given the diagnosis of postoperative PID. She is admitted to the Gynecology floor and started on triple antibiotics. Three hours after admission, you are consulted because her abdominal pain is increasing, her temperature has increased to 102.3°F, her blood pressure is 80/40, and her heart rate is in the 130s. Her abdomen is diffusely tender with rebound in all quadrants. You review an upright abdominal film taken on admission (Figure 116). What is the most likely etiology of her symptoms and signs?

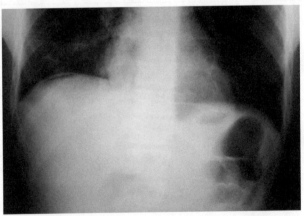

Figure 116 • Image provided by Departments of Radiology and Obstetrics & Gynecology, University of California, San Francisco.

A. Postoperative PID
B. Endomyometritis
C. Appendicitis
D. Ureteral injury
E. Bowel injury

117. A 62-year-old woman is admitted for exploratory laparotomy and debulking procedure for likely ovarian cancer. Upon entering the abdomen, there is bulky disease on every peritoneal surface and surrounding much of the bowel and omentum (a "peek and shriek" case). No further surgical intervention is undertaken, and the patient is closed and subsequently admitted postoperatively to the gynecologic oncology service for her first round of chemotherapy. What should her chemotherapeutic regimen include?

A. CHOP (cyclophosphamide, doxorubicin, oncovin, prednisone)
B. Taxol and carboplatin
C. Melphalan
D. Etoposide and cisplatin
E. CMF (cyclophosphamide, methotrexate, fluorouracil)

118. A 37-year-old woman is undergoing a TAH-BSO for chronic pelvic pain from stage IV endometriosis. There is extensive dissection to free the left adnexa from the bowel and from the pelvic sidewalls. Identification of the ureter on the left side is adequate, but the right ureter is difficult to identify above the pelvic brim. At one point in the procedure, there is a question of right ureteral injury. After the specimen is removed, indigo-carmine dye is given intravenously and spills out of the right ureter approximately 4 cm above the pelvic brim. The distal portion is easily identified and there is no obviously missing portion. What is the best repair for this injury?

A. End-to-end reanastomosis
B. End-to-side reanastomosis
C. Ureteral reimplantation into the bladder dome
D. Ureteral reimplantation into the contralateral ureter
E. Cannot be repaired—place nephrostomy tube

119. A 47-year-old woman undergoes a radical hysterectomy and bilateral salpingo-oophorectomy for Stage Ib cervical carcinoma. At the beginning of the procedure, compression stockings and pneumoboots are placed for deep vein thrombosis (DVT) prophylaxis. During the procedure, she has an estimated blood loss of 750 cc. In addition to pneumoboots, which of the following is commonly used for DVT prophylaxis in postoperative patients with cancer?

A. Coumadin
B. Heparin SQ 5000 units TID
C. Low-molecular-weight (LMW) heparin SQ 40 units QD
D. LMW heparin SQ 40 units BID
E. Anticoagulation is not given postoperatively

120. A 32-year-old G_0 woman is undergoing laparoscopy for evaluation of her infertility. A hysterosalpingogram (HSG) showed spillage from the left fallopian tube, but only partial filling on the right. The patient has no history of pelvic pain or dysmenorrhea. In addition, she has regular menses and a positive LH spike on day 13 of her cycle. On entering the abdomen, you notice extensive pelvic adhesions and a 3- to 4-cm endometrioma on the right ovary. The right adnexa is adherent to the right pelvic sidewall. When the uterus is injected with indigo-carmine dye, there is spillage from both fallopian tubes—first from the left and then a small trickle from the right. What is the etiology of this patient's infertility?

A. Chronic PID leading to lack of tubal patency
B. Endometriosis leading to lack of tubal patency
C. Endometriosis leading to ovarian dysfunction
D. Endometriosis with uncertain pathophysiology
E. Uncertain etiology leading to lack of tubal patency

121. A 36-year-old G_0 woman presents for operative hysteroscopy and resection of an intrauterine fibroid, which is the presumed cause of her infertility. During the case, the uterus is sounded to 7 cm. During dilation, you notice that dilation is quite difficult until suddenly the 7 French dilator passes easily, but to a distance of 10 cm. Presumably, you have perforated the uterus. What is the next step in this patient's management?

A. Continue with the case
B. Proceed to exploratory laparotomy
C. Continue with the case and treat with antibiotics
D. Follow vital signs and order a pelvic US
E. As most of these perforations are not associated with morbidity, allow the patient to go home

122. A 26-year-old G_1 woman with pregestational type 1 diabetes mellitus presents to labor and delivery for planned induction at 39 weeks GA. Her first prenatal visit was at 7 weeks GA. An US at that time was consistent with a certain LMP. The patient has been monitoring her blood sugars and self-administering insulin since the age of 13, enjoyed good glycemic control before and during this pregnancy, and brings meticulous records to each prenatal visit. An US last week showed growth consistent with dates and normal amniotic fluid. Biophysical profile score was 10/10. On admission, the patient's blood pressure is 105/80. Urine dipstick shows trace glucose and no protein. She is without complaint, but after seeing the impact of pregnancy on her blood sugars, she is concerned about how her disease will affect her labor, delivery, and recovery. How are this patient's insulin requirements most likely to change in the intrapartum and postpartum periods as compared to her third trimester of pregnancy?

A. Increased intrapartum, increased postpartum
B. Increased intrapartum, decreased postpartum
C. Decreased intrapartum, increased postpartum
D. Decreased intrapartum, decreased postpartum
E. Decreased intrapartum, no change postpartum

The next two questions (items 123 and 124) correspond to the following vignette.

A 23-year-old G_1 woman at 33 weeks GA is sent from the clinic to labor and delivery for evaluation of preeclampsia. She was healthy prior to pregnancy, and did not have any elevated blood pressures or proteinuria in her pregnancy until this afternoon. When she presented for her routine prenatal visit (after missing her last two appointments), her blood pressure was 150/98 and urine dipstick revealed 2+ proteinuria. She denied symptoms of preeclampsia. On arrival to labor and delivery, a 24-hour urine collection is started, blood pressures are carefully monitored, and an US is performed.

123. Which of the following, if true, would classify her preeclampsia as severe, rather than mild?

  A. Blood pressures are measured in the range 145–150/95–100
  B. 1500 mg protein is collected over 24 hours
  C. Ultrasonography estimates fetal weight at the 13th percentile
  D. The patient is experiencing swelling of her hands
  E. The patient is experiencing right upper quadrant pain and tenderness, and has an elevated aspartate transaminase (AST) level

124. Based on the initial assessment, mild preeclampsia is suspected in this patient. A plan to administer corticosteroids and initiate expectant management is discussed with her. Immediately after this discussion, the laboratory calls to report AST = 220 U/L, ALT = 190 U/L, and platelets = 75,000/μL. How does this information change your management of this patient?

  A. No change in management
  B. Immediate cesarean delivery
  C. Initiate tocolysis to allow time for 48 hours of corticosteroids
  D. Continue corticosteroids and move toward vaginal delivery
  E. Continue expectant management, but begin magnesium sulfate

End of set

---

125. A 28-year-old G_5P_3 woman presents to labor and delivery 20 minutes following vaginal delivery of a full-term infant in the ambulance en route to the hospital. She told the paramedics that she had ruptured her membranes 6 hours before calling 911. The patient is admitted and a secondary vaginal laceration is repaired. During the exam and repair, multiple vesicular vulvar and perineal lesions are noted. The patient is very uncooperative and refuses to answer questions about her obstetrical or medical history. Review of her prenatal chart is notable for culture-confirmed herpes simplex virus (HSV-2) 5 days prior; no other antenatal issues are noted. The pediatrics service is now attempting to assess the risk of disseminated neonatal herpes infection. Which of the following, if found in the patient's prenatal chart, would increase your concern for disseminated HSV infection?

  A. The patient reported three outbreaks of lesions prior to this pregnancy
  B. The current outbreak began in the second trimester
  C. The patient has a history of oral HSV-1 infection since childhood
  D. A maternal anti-HSV IgG titer drawn 5 days ago was negative
  E. Acyclovir was started at 36 weeks GA

> **The next three questions (items 126, 127, and 128) correspond to the following vignette.**

Thirty-six hours after delivery of a viable female infant, a 32-year-old G₂P₁ woman develops a temperature of 38.6°C and shaking chills. Her labor was induced at 42 0/7 weeks GA with oxytocin. The first stage of labor lasted 37 hours, the second stage lasted 4.5 hours, and the third stage lasted 24 minutes. Artificial rupture of membranes was performed 19 hours prior to delivery. An episiotomy was performed with a third-degree extension. Estimated blood loss was 450 cc. The patient received an epidural for analgesia. She was afebrile during her labor. Her prenatal labs were all normal and included a negative GBS culture and HIV test.

126. What is the most common puerperal infection after a vaginal delivery?

   A. Infected vaginal hematoma
   B. Endomyometritis
   C. Thrombophlebitis
   D. Pyelonephritis
   E. Pneumonia

127. Which of the following tests should be performed first?

   A. Chest X-ray
   B. Bimanual exam
   C. Pelvic US
   D. Lower-extremity Doppler
   E. Sputum culture

128. An aerobic culture reveals gram-negative rods. Which of the following is the most likely to be the etiologic organism in a puerperal infection after vaginal birth in this culture?

   A. *Staphylococcus epidermidis*
   B. *Escherichia coli*
   C. *Enterococcus species*
   D. *Bacteroides fragilis*
   E. *Chlamydia trachomatis*

End of set

> **The next two questions (items 129 and 130) correspond to the following vignette.**

A 22-year-old G₁P₁ woman is 14 hours after a vaginal delivery of a healthy baby girl. The patient has tried to breastfeed, but thus far is discouraged because she has not produced very much breast milk. You encourage her and discuss with her the physiology of breastfeeding as well as its long-term benefits.

129. Compared to mature milk, colostrum contains:

A. More fat
B. Fewer minerals
C. More protein
D. More sugar
E. The exact same contents, but in a more concentrated form

130. The release of which hormone is responsible for the milk "let-down" reflex?

A. Estrogen
B. Prolactin
C. Oxytocin
D. Placental lactogen
E. Stimulactogen

End of set

---

131. You are asked by your chief resident to counsel a new mother regarding breast-feeding versus formula feeding for her new baby. Before going to talk to the patient, you review the literature on the benefits of breastfeeding. You tell her that the benefits of breastfeeding her infant will include which of the following?

A. Increased childhood allergies
B. Decreased infantile ear infections
C. Decreased postpartum maternal weight loss
D. More rapid weight gain for her infant
E. Decreased rates of autism

132. A 28-year-old G_1P_0 woman at 38 1/7 weeks GA with poorly controlled gestational diabetes has been completely dilated and pushing for more than 2 hours. You are called for the delivery and notice prolonged crowning of the head followed by the "turtle" sign. After delivery of the head, you apply gentle downward traction on the head but the shoulders do not easily deliver. What is your next step to deliver this infant?

A. Persistent strong downward traction of the head
B. Attempt a vacuum-assisted vaginal delivery
C. Attempt a forceps-assisted vaginal delivery
D. Sharply flex the maternal hips and apply moderate suprapubic pressure
E. Apply forceful pressure on the uterine fundus

133. A 30-year-old G_1 woman at 32 3/7 weeks GA presents to labor and delivery with uterine contractions and cervical change consistent with preterm labor. She is admitted and placed on magnesium sulfate for tocolysis. What is the most likely benefit from this tocolysis?

A. Prolonging pregnancy for an additional 48 hours to allow for treatment with antibiotics
B. Prolonging pregnancy for an additional 48 hours to allow for treatment with steroids
C. Stopping uterine contractions and increasing the likelihood of a term delivery
D. Decreasing the rate of maternal and neonatal seizures
E. There is no benefit of magnesium sulfate tocolysis in this patient

134. A 29-year-old G_2P_1 woman at 28 2/7 weeks GA presents with a single episode of bright red, painless vaginal bleeding soaking a large towel. She denies uterine contractions, loss of fluid, trauma, or recent intercourse, and describes normal fetal movement. Abdominal exam reveals a nontender uterus. Speculum exam is notable for a moderate amount of bright red blood in the vagina and a visually closed, normal-appearing cervix. Fetal heart tracing is reassuring and no uterine contractions are demonstrated on tocometry. US is obtained (Figure 134). What is the most likely etiology for antepartum hemorrhage in this patient?

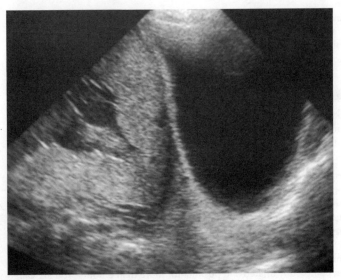

Figure 134 • Image provided by Departments of Radiology and Obstetrics & Gynecology, University of California, San Francisco.

    A. Placental abruption
    B. Placenta previa
    C. Cervical cancer
    D. Preterm labor
    E. Hemorrhoids

135. You are seeing a 28-year-old G_2P_1 woman at 37 1/7 weeks GA with multiple complaints including shortness of breath, fatigue, sneezing, congestion, nausea, and vomiting. Her blood pressure is 103/77, her pulse is 110, her respiratory rate is 22, and room air saturation is 90%. The patient's urinalysis reveals 3+ ketones and a specific gravity of 1.030. You perform a physical exam and several laboratory tests including a CBC, electrolytes, and arterial blood gas. Of the following results, which is the most concerning?

    A. Blood urea nitrogen of 4 and creatinine of 0.5
    B. WBC count of 15 million/mL
    C. Arterial blood gas with a P_{CO_2} of 44 mm Hg
    D. Hematocrit of 33%
    E. Mean corpuscular volume (MCV) of 78

136. A 34-year-old G_3P_0 woman at 18 3/7 weeks GA without complaints was sent to labor and delivery by the US department because on US her cervix was 1.5 cm long with funneling. She notes fetal movement and denies contractions, leakage of amniotic fluid, and vaginal bleeding. The patient reports that she has a history of cervical dysplasia treated with conization. On her chart, you note a history of two second trimester losses occurring without painful contractions. The FHR tracing is reactive, and the tocometer shows no uterine activity. Her cervix is closed at the external os, 1.5 cm long, and 50% effaced. An US image of her cervix is obtained (Figure 136). You diagnose her with incompetent cervix and recommend which of the following measures?

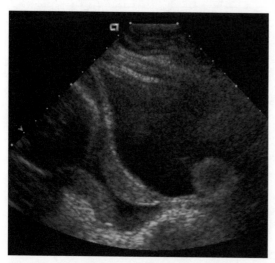

Figure 136 · Image provided by Departments of Radiology and Obstetrics & Gynecology, University of California, San Francisco.

A. Bedrest and betamethasone
B. IV antibiotics
C. Trendelenburg position
D. Cervical cerclage
E. Tocolysis

137. A 22-year-old G_1P_0 woman at 37 3/7 weeks GA is referred for elevated blood pressure in the clinic. Her blood pressure is 147/93. Her urinalysis is significant for 3+ protein. The patient has been seeing "spots" in her visual field since she woke up this morning. You decide to admit her to the labor unit and induce her labor. You examine her cervix and monitor the fetus and the patient's contractions. Her fetus has a reactive FHR tracing, she is not having contractions, and her cervix is unfavorable. You plan to use PGE_1 (misoprostol) for cervical ripening. You check the amniotic fluid index (AFI), which is 7 cm. You obtain further maternal medical history and decide that it is unsafe to use misoprostol. What are the maternal contraindications to prostaglandins?

A. Hypertension and asthma
B. Asthma and glaucoma
C. Hypertension and uterine contractions every 4 minutes
D. Hypertension and an AFI less than 10 cm
E. Glaucoma and preeclampsia

138. You are managing the labor of a 25-year-old G_2P_1 woman with preeclampsia. She is in spontaneous active labor and making adequate progress with uterine contractions every 3 to 4 minutes. She is currently 8 cm dilated and 0 station. The FHR tracing reveals minimal variability (Figure 138). You perform a fetal scalp stimulation. The FHR tracing reveals no acceleration in response. You then decide to perform a fetal scalp pH. Which of the values below is matched with the appropriate action?

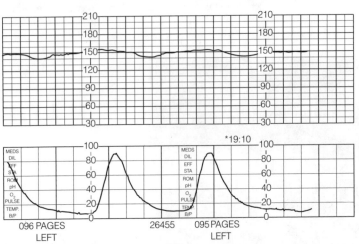

Figure 138 • Reproduced with permission from Callahan T. Blueprints Obstetrics & Gynecology. 3rd ed. Blackwell, 2004: Fig. 4-6 B, p. 37.

- **A.** Fetal scalp pH 7.30—expectant management
- **B.** Fetal scalp pH 7.10—resample
- **C.** Fetal scalp pH 7.15—expectant management
- **D.** Fetal scalp pH 7.55—cesarean section
- **E.** Fetal scalp pH 7.22—cesarean section

The next two questions (items 139 and 140) correspond to the following vignette.

A 26-year-old G_2P_1 woman at 40 2/7 weeks GA has been in the active phase of labor for 7 hours. She is receiving a Pitocin infusion of 16 mU/min for uterine contractions and is contracting every $2\frac{1}{2}$ to 4 minutes. Her pain is controlled via epidural analgesia. The FHR tracing falls to the 90 beats/min range (Figure 139). Despite maternal repositioning and delivery of O_2 by face mask, the deceleration persists for $4\frac{1}{2}$ minutes. You perform a vaginal exam and find that the patient's cervix is completely dilated and the fetal vertex is occiput anterior and −1 station with no other findings.

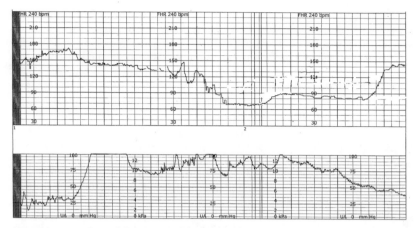

Figure 139 · Image provided by Department of Obstetrics & Gynecology, University of California, San Francisco.

139. What is the most likely cause for the prolonged deceleration?

A. Cord compression
B. Placenta previa
C. Tetanic contraction
D. Cord prolapse
E. Precipitous delivery

140. Considering the most likely cause of the FHR deceleration, which of the following is the most appropriate course of action?

A. Emergent cesarean section
B. Forceps-assisted vaginal delivery
C. Stop the Pitocin infusion and administer terbutaline subcutaneously
D. Elevation of the fetal vertex
E. Scalp pH sampling

End of set

141. A 23-year-old G_2P_1 woman at 41 2/7 weeks GA reports a history of a normal spontaneous vaginal delivery at 35 weeks. She is in active labor and her labor course has been protracted. Currently, she has been at 7 cm for 4 hours. You augmented her labor with amniotomy and oxytocin. An IUPC was placed 6 hours ago, and her uterine contractions are now occurring every 3 minutes, each approximately 70 Montevideo units. The FHR tracing has a baseline in the 120s with moderate variability, rare accelerations, and occasional variable decelerations. Which of the following is the appropriate next step in this patient's management?

A. Perform a cesarean section for fetal indications
B. Perform a cesarean section for active-phase arrest with adequate forces
C. Perform a cesarean section for prolonged second stage
D. Perform a cesarean section for active-phase arrest without adequate forces
E. Perform a cesarean section but only after 3 more hours of active-phase arrest

142. A 17-year-old G_1P_0 woman at 34 weeks GA by LMP presents with decreased urine output, dyspnea, and blood pressure of 145/110. Her urinalysis shows 2+ proteinuria. You diagnose her with preeclampsia and admit her to the ward for labor induction. Additionally, you administer a 4-g loading dose followed by a 2-g/h infusion of magnesium sulfate for seizure prophylaxis. While checking on the patient later in the day, you notice that her magnesium sulfate drip is running at 10 g/h rather than 2 g/h. You quickly stop the IV and check the patient's magnesium level. As magnesium levels rise, which is the first side effect seen?

A. Loss of deep tendon reflexes
B. Cardiac arrest
C. Seizures
D. Pulmonary suppression
E. Cortical blindness

143. A 39-year-old G_3P_2 woman at 32 weeks GA is hospitalized for treatment of a solitary pulmonary nodule, which was confirmed on biopsy to be primary adenocarcinoma of the lung. Which of the following is true regarding cancer in pregnancy?

A. Metastasis to the fetus occurs
B. Chemotherapy is contraindicated throughout pregnancy
C. Survival is higher when breast cancer is diagnosed during pregnancy compared to the nonpregnant state
D. Radiation treatment is a recommended therapy in pregnancy
E. Termination of pregnancy improves cancer prognosis

144. A 15-year-old G_0 female is undergoing exploratory laparotomy for an 8-cm complex left ovarian mass that was diagnosed last week when she presented to the ED with symptoms concerning for ovarian torsion. Doppler US revealed no evidence of acute torsion, and the patient was discharged home with strict torsion precautions as well as a consultation appointment with gynecologic oncology. Which of the following tumors is accurately paired with the appropriate tumor marker?

A. Choriocarcinoma and alpha-fetoprotein (AFP)
B. Dysgerminoma and AFP
C. Embryonal carcinoma and hCG and AFP
D. Endodermal sinus tumor and CA-125
E. Immature teratoma and hCG

The next two questions (items 145 and 146) correspond to the following vignette.

A 40 year-old woman is admitted from the ED with severe menorrhagia and symptomatic anemia (hematocrit = 15) for observation and blood transfusion. An US is obtained (Figure 145).

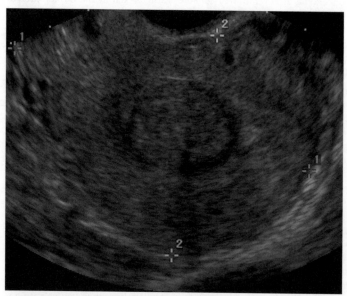

Figure 145 · Image provided by Departments of Radiology and Obstetrics & Gynecology, University of California, San Francisco.

145. What is her diagnosis and the likely source of her menorrhagia?

   A. Cervical cancer
   B. Submucosal fibroid
   C. Ovarian cancer
   D. Endometrial polyp
   E. Tubo-ovarian abscess (TOA)

146. Given her diagnosis, which of the following is an appropriate treatment option?

   A. Thermal balloon ablation
   B. LEEP
   C. Cone biopsy
   D. Hysteroscopic resection
   E. Total abdominal hysterectomy with bilateral salpingo-oophorectomy (TAH-BSO)

End of set

147. You are called to see a 54-year-old patient who is postoperative day 2 status post an uncomplicated total abdominal hysterectomy (TAH) for fibroids. The patient now has a temperature of 100.8°F. She is on Demerol and an antiemetic and has no significant past medical history. You arrive to find an obese patient in no apparent distress. She reports feeling slightly warm but denies cough, shortness of breath, pain, difficulty ambulating, dysuria or hematuria, problems with her incision, or passage of flatus since surgery. She has ambulated once today after removal of her Foley catheter, stating she was too tired to do more. On exam, her incision appears clean, dry, and intact, with staples in place, and her abdomen is soft and nontender. Bowel sounds are decreased but present in all four quadrants. Her lungs are clear but breath sounds are decreased at the bilateral bases. Her calves are nontender. What is the most likely diagnosis and appropriate management of her postoperative fever?

    A. Urinary tract infection—initiate antibiotic therapy
    B. Wound cellulitis—initiate antibiotic therapy
    C. Atelectasis—incentive spirometry, ambulation, and observation of temperatures
    D. Deep vein thrombosis (DVT)—lower-extremity Doppler US
    E. Postoperative infection—check blood cultures, urine culture, and chest x-ray; initiate antibiotic therapy

148. A 37-year-old woman is 6 hours status post an exploratory laparotomy and right salpingo-oophorectomy for a large adnexal cyst involving so much of her ovary that a cystectomy could not safely be performed without resulting in a large amount of bleeding. The estimated blood loss (EBL) from the procedure was 1000 mL. When you perform a postoperative check on her now, you notice that she is lying in bed and appears pale. Her blood pressure is 100/62, pulse is 132, respiratory rate is 16, and temperature and oxygen saturation are both normal. The patient's urine output has been approximately 280 mL since her surgery, but over the last hour, she has made only 15 mL of urine. She reports that her pain is controlled, but when you palpate her abdomen, it is somewhat distended and surprisingly tender to the patient. You hear very faint and rare bowel sounds. Exam of her dressing reveals a large amount of bloody drainage, but the incision and fascia are intact. What is the most appropriate next step in management of this patient?

    A. Abdominal X-ray
    B. Remove her Foley catheter and have her void spontaneously
    C. Check a stat hemoglobin/hematocrit
    D. Exploratory laparotomy
    E. Remove her staples and probe her wound

149. A 49-year-old G_1P_1 woman is postoperative day 2 following a total abdominal hysterectomy (TAH) for chronic pelvic pain and large fibroids. Her surgery was made difficult by dense pelvic and bowel adhesions due to endometriosis, requiring extensive lysis of adhesions. You are called to see her for severe nausea and vomiting that is refractory to antiemetics. She had minimal bowel sounds on exam this morning and denied passage of flatus. At that time, she had only minimal nausea and her diet was advanced to clear liquids. The patient's medications include a morphine sulfate patient-controlled analgesia (PCA) device, which she has used liberally since surgery, as well as ondansetron for nausea and vomiting. She has ambulated only once since this morning. On exam, she has rare bowel sounds and her abdomen is mildly diffusely, tender to palpation, distended, and tympanic, but without rebound or guarding. Her incision is clean, dry, and intact, with staples in place. You obtain an abdominal film (Figure 149). What is the best treatment for this patient?

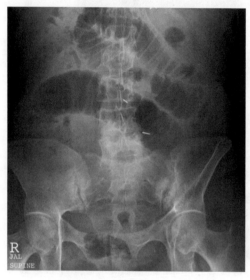

Figure 149 • Image provided by Departments of Radiology and Obstetrics & Gynecology, University of California, San Francisco.

A. Advance diet as tolerated
B. NPO, IV hydration
C. Take back to the operating room for exploratory laparotomy
D. NPO, nasogastric tube
E. Milk of magnesia

150. A 57-year-old G_0 postmenopausal woman is undergoing exploratory laparotomy, total abdominal hysterectomy, bilateral salpingo-oophorectomy, and staging for suspected ovarian malignancy. The patient originally presented complaining of abdominal bloating for 6 months along with an 8-lb weight loss achieved without dieting. A pelvic US revealed massive ascites and bilateral 6-cm complex adnexal masses (Figure 150). Which of the following statements is true regarding the major types of ovarian tumors?

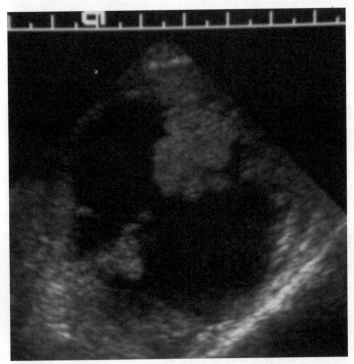

Figure 150 • Image provided by Departments of Radiology and Obstetrics & Gynecology, University of California, San Francisco.

A. Germ cell tumors are the most common
B. Sex-cord stromal tumors include granulosa-theca and Sertoli-Leydig tumors
C. Epithelial cell tumors are more frequent among women in their twenties
D. Germ cell tumors are more frequent among women in their late fifties
E. Germ cell tumors include mucinous and endometrioid tumors

Answer Key

101.	B	118.	A	135.	C
102.	A	119.	B	136.	D
103.	C	120.	D	137.	B
104.	D	121.	D	138.	A
105.	C	122.	D	139.	C
106.	E	123.	E	140.	C
107.	B	124.	D	141.	B
108.	C	125.	D	142.	A
109.	B	126.	B	143.	A
110.	E	127.	B	144.	C
111.	B	128.	B	145.	B
112.	B	129.	C	146.	D
113.	C	130.	C	147.	C
114.	A	131.	B	148.	C
115.	B	132.	D	149.	B
116.	E	133.	B	150.	B
117.	B	134.	B		

101. **B.** A low forceps delivery is defined as at least +2 station, meaning that the fetal skull is at least 2 cm below the ischial spines. An outlet forceps is when the fetal scalp is visible without separating the labia. A mid forceps is when the head is between 0 and +2 station and engaged. Anything above a mid forceps is a high forceps, which is no longer practiced in the United States because of its association with fetal injury.

A. Adequate anesthesia is necessary for an operative vaginal delivery. Often it will consist of an epidural, but it can also be a pudendal block or (rarely) spinal anesthesia.

C. Fetal macrosomia is a relative contraindication to operative vaginal delivery because it is associated with shoulder dystocia, which is associated with higher risk of perinatal morbidity and mortality. However, this fetus does not meet any criteria of fetal macrosomia, which ranges in definition from 4000 g to the most commonly used 4500-g threshold. If anything, the fact that the patient successfully delivered a prior fetus who was thought to be larger than this fetus is reassuring.

D. The fetal position is LOA, so it meets the criteria for a nonrotation. While knowledge of the fetal position is imperative for operative vaginal delivery, the actual position itself is rarely a contraindication. However, it may change the skill level needed from the clinician and the designation of the type of forceps delivery. For example, if the fetal position is LOT, to perform a forceps delivery, a 90° rotation will need to be performed. LOT position would be a contraindication for clinicians not trained to perform rotations.

E. Maternal exhaustion is actually an indication for elective operative vaginal delivery.

102. **A.** Classically, to diagnose active-phase arrest of labor or failure to progress in labor, adequate forces of labor must be demonstrated. The strength of contractions can be measured with an IUPC, as the external tocometer simply measures the frequency and duration of contractions. The units used most commonly to describe the forces of labor are Montevideo units. They are calculated by measuring the difference between the baseline and peak intrauterine pressures of the individual contractions summed over a 10-minute period. Adequate forces are greater than or equal to 180 to 200 Montevideo units. Failure to progress in labor is usually defined when (1) adequate forces are demonstrated and (2) the patient has no change in cervical dilation or station over a period of 2 hours in the active phase. At this point, cesarean delivery is commonly offered. Of note, one recent study suggests that waiting for 4 rather than 2 hours may lead to another 60% of patients delivering vaginally (Rouse DJ, Owen J, Savage KG, Hauth JC. Active phase labor arrest: revisiting the 2-hour minimum. Obstet Gynecol 2001;98:550–554).

B. On the Friedman curve, a cervical dilation of at least 1 cm per hour is expected in the active phase, which is actually the 5th percentile of cervical change. That is, 95% of all patients will dilate at 1 cm per hour or faster.

C. Commonly, if the forces of labor as measured are inadequate, oxytocin is begun and increased until contractions are considered adequate. Many patients will achieve adequate labor on their own and will not need oxytocin augmentation. Alternatively, if a patient is not making adequate progress, she is often begun on oxytocin augmentation prior to receiving the IUPC.

D. Active-phase arrest of labor is diagnosed when, in the setting of adequate forces of labor as measured by an IUPC, no change in dilation or station occurs during a 2-hour period.

E. The duration of the active phase of labor differs between multiparous and nulliparous patients. The total length is not actually used to make the diagnosis of failure to progress. One reason for this is that a patient with inadequate labor may undergo slow cervical change for several hours before augmentation is begun, thus increasing the total length of labor.

103. C. Late and variable FHR decelerations are generally a sign of acute decrease in oxygen, which leads to vagal stimulation and a decrease in the FHR. The decelerations described here are associated with contractions, begin after the contraction begins, and end after the contraction is over. This is a description of late decelerations, which are associated with uteroplacental insufficiency. Uteroplacental insufficiency itself can be caused by decreased maternal perfusion of the uterus secondary to anemia, hypoxia, or hypotension, as well as by poor gas exchange across the placenta secondary to increased placental resistance or abruption.

A. Early decelerations begin and end with contractions and are thought to be due to fetal head compression.

B. Variable decelerations are not necessarily associated with contractions. They are sudden in onset, and the FHR reaches its nadir within 15 to 30 seconds. These decelerations are thought to occur secondary to umbilical cord compression.

D. Late decelerations are not caused by head compression.

E. A nuchal cord—that is, an umbilical cord that is wrapped around the fetal neck—is seen in 10% to 15% of pregnancies. As the fetus descends, the nuchal cord can be pulled and compressed, leading to variable decelerations.

104. D. Uterine atony is the most common etiology of postpartum hemorrhage. This patient has multiple risk factors for postpartum hemorrhage due to uterine atony, including chorioamnionitis, use of magnesium sulfate, and a macrosomic fetus. In addition to uterine massage, uterine atony is treated with uterotonic agents such as oxytocin, $PGF_{2\alpha}$ (Hemabate), and methylergonovine (Methergine).

A. A cervical laceration is not an uncommon cause of a postpartum hemorrhage. This patient has one risk factor for cervical laceration—a macrosomic fetus. Other risk factors include a fast labor and pushing against a cervix that is not fully dilated. Cervical laceration is still much less likely than uterine atony.

B. A vaginal laceration, particularly one into the pelvic sidewall, can bleed quite impressively. Vaginal lacerations are more likely in the setting of an operative vaginal delivery.

C. Ruptured hemorrhoidal vessels are an uncommon source of blood loss after delivery.

E. Retained POCs such as a placental cotyledon or a succenturiate lobe may lead to uterine atony and postpartum hemorrhage. On exam, this patient's placenta was intact, and there was no evidence of a succenturiate lobe. In this setting, uterine exploration for retained POCs is indicated only after all other treatments have failed.

105. **C.** The liver transaminases, AST and alanine transaminase (ALT), are commonly checked as a part of routine preeclampsia labs. Substantial elevation—particularly twice the normal level—is consistent with HELLP syndrome, in the absence of other hepatic pathology. HELLP syndrome is a severe variant of preeclampsia and always demands delivery regardless of GA.

A. Creatinine is essential to assess renal function. Creatinine levels in pregnancy should be low, certainly less than 0.7, because the glomerular filtration rate (GFR) is increased. A mildly elevated creatinine level is often abnormal. However, a creatinine abnormality is not a part of HELLP syndrome.

B. The hematocrit can identify the degree of hemoconcentration, which is another feature of preeclampsia. With HELLP, the hematocrit should be falling secondary to hemolysis. Because of the two effects of hemoconcentration and hemolysis, better diagnostic tests for hemolysis are lactate dehydrogenase (LDH) or peripheral blood smear.

D. Uric acid levels have been noted to be elevated in patients with preeclampsia, but have not been formally added to the diagnostic criteria or even the screening criteria. One study did show that this measure can be used to screen for preeclampsia among patients with renal disease and/or chronic hypertension who have normal baseline serum uric acid levels. In these high-risk patients, a uric acid level that is increasing or that is higher than 6.0 is a good screening tool for preeclampsia.

E. A low platelet count (less than 150,000) is needed for the diagnosis of HELLP syndrome. However, this finding can be misleading because 8% of pregnant women at term may have a platelet count between 100,000 and 150,000.

106. **E.** Twin pregnancies can be dizygotic (two initial zygotes) or monozygotic (one initial zygote that splits into two at some point). Dizygotic twins will always be dichorionic and diamnionic (di/di)—two placentas and two amniotic cavities. Monozygotic twins can be di/di, mono/di, mono/mono, or conjoined (known by laypersons as "Siamese"), depending on when the zygote splits. At delivery, twin pregnancies can present in a variety of ways. Each fetus can be cephalic (head first), breech (buttocks first), or transverse, creating nine possible presentations. If the presenting fetus is cephalic, and the twins are concordant, a TOL with cephalic delivery or breech extraction of the second twin is reasonable.

A. Vaginal delivery of a breech-presenting twin followed by a cephalic twin is usually not allowed. In addition to the usual risks of delivering the breech-presenting twin, there is a risk of interlocking twins, wherein the second twin's head comes through the pelvis before the first twin's head.

B. After the delivery of the first twin, the uterus rapidly decreases in size, which increases the risk for abruption of the second twin's placenta. Augmentation with high-dose oxytocin is likely to increase the risk of abruption and tetanic contractions and, therefore, is contraindicated. Classically, the occurrence of an undiagnosed twin is the reason oxytocin is not given until after delivery of the placenta.

C. Forceps should never be applied when the cervix is not fully dilated.

D. If both twins are cephalic presenting, there is no indication for cesarean delivery.

107. **B.** The decision to attempt a TOL in the setting of a breech presentation is one that needs careful counseling. Common requirements include a fetus between 2500 and 4000 g, a flexed fetal head, no fetal or uterine anomalies, and an adequate maternal pelvis as determined by clinical or CT pelvimetry. A recent prospective, randomized, multicenter trial demonstrated that women randomized to TOL had higher rates of fetal trauma. However, because this trial included centers that did not have fetal monitoring and did not use CT pelvimetry, it has been criticized. Because the diameters of the head are minimized with flexion, the head of a breech-presenting fetus undergoing a TOL should be flexed to avoid head entrapment.

A. Generally, the fetus undergoing breech delivery should be less than 4000 g or not macrosomic. Some practitioners will use a lower cutoff of 3800 g because of the inaccuracy of US and Leopold maneuvers.

C. While it is frequently suggested to the patient that she have adequate anesthesia, often via an epidural, lack of epidural anesthesia is not an absolute contraindication to a vaginal breech delivery. However, because of the likely need for piper forceps and possible need for emergent cesarean delivery, patients undergoing a TOL for a breech presentation are recommended to have epidural anesthesia.

D. While a prior vaginal delivery, considered a "proven pelvis," is desirable, the absence of such is not a contraindication.

E. Few studies have examined breech vaginal delivery after prior cesarean section. In those rare studies conducted on this issue, there was no obvious increase in complications other than those from a breech vaginal delivery.

108. **C.** Betamethasone or dexamethasone is given to patients between 24 and 34 weeks GA at acute risk for preterm delivery. Several prospective, randomized, controlled trials (conducted as early as 1972) showed that these agents decrease the risk of respiratory distress syndrome and increase the rate of survival. Later studies demonstrated decreased rates of intraventricular hemorrhage and necrotizing enterocolitis.

A, D. This patient is in preterm labor (i.e., regular uterine contractions that cause cervical change) and should be tocolyzed to prevent preterm delivery. Magnesium sulfate is commonly used for tocolysis in preterm labor. Other agents used for tocolysis include terbutaline, ritodrine, indomethacin, and nifedipine. The principal benefit of these tocolytic agents has been to increase the length of pregnancy by 48 hours. Fortunately, that is the amount of time necessary to gain the benefits from betamethasone. While tocolysis is an important aspect of this patient's care, administration of antenatal corticosteroids to promote fetal lung maturity is more important. Terbutaline is another tocolytic agent.

B. Erythromycin is used in conjunction with ampicillin in patients with preterm premature rupture of the membranes to promote prolonged latency period (time from rupture of membranes to delivery). However, erythromycin is not commonly used for prophylaxis in patients with intact membranes, like the patient in this case.

E. IV penicillin is commonly used in preterm labor or term labor in women who are documented GBS carriers. Its widespread use has decreased the rate of neonatal sepsis. However, its effectiveness in a preterm patient pales in comparison to that of betamethasone.

---

109. | **B.** There is evidence from a large, randomized, controlled trial in patients with PROM at term. Of note in examining that study's results, "premature" refers to rupture of membranes prior to the initiation of uterine contractions; in contrast, "preterm" refers to rupture of membranes occurring in a fetus of less than 37 weeks GA. In that investigation, patients who underwent immediate induction of labor with either oxytocin or prostaglandins delivered sooner than those who underwent expectant management. The length of labor, rate of operative delivery, and use of epidural anesthesia were roughly the same for both groups. The rates of maternal infection were higher in the expectant management group. Thus the most commonly recommended course of management for patients with term PROM is induction of labor.

A, E. It is not common practice to discharge patients with term PROM to home. However, some patients strongly prefer spontaneous onset of labor and will want expectant management at home. In these patients, frequent temperature checks and daily visits to the hospital for fetal nonstress tests are an important component of management. No protocol suggests implementing this management for longer than 72 hours, at which time induction should be strongly suggested.

C. In patients with preterm PROM, antibiotics are given to increase the time until labor ensues. At term, antibiotics are used prophylactically only in patients who are GBS positive.

D. Betamethasone is only used in patients until 34 weeks GA.

---

110. | **E.** The most common cause of ambiguous genitalia is congenital adrenal hyperplasia (CAH). Three common enzyme deficiencies can lead to CAH: (1) 3-β-hydroxy-steroid dehydrogenase, (2) 11-β-hydroxylase, and, most commonly, (3) 21-hydroxylase. 21-Hydroxylase deficiency leads to accumulation of 17-hydroxyprogesterone and a deficiency of cortisol and the mineralocorticoids. Testosterone is slightly elevated, but progesterone and estrogen levels are usually normal. As a consequence, male fetuses usually have an entirely normal appearance, but female newborns may have ambiguous genitalia. Medical treatment involves replacement of the missing steroid hormones.

A. Corrective surgery should be deferred for at least several months to allow for adjustment to medical therapy, but should be performed before the child can remember the gender confusion. Parents may push to have the surgery as soon as possible.

B. Estradiol is usually normal.

C. Progesterone will be either normal or slightly elevated, and does not need replacement.

D. Testosterone is likely elevated in this newborn, leading to the ambiguous genitalia.

111. **B.** This patient has experienced a prolapsed umbilical cord, which is an obstetric emergency requiring immediate cesarean delivery. In the setting of an emergent cesarean delivery, it is reasonable to utilize spinal anesthesia as long as it can be administered quickly and there is no evidence of abruption, uterine rupture, or ongoing fetal hypoxia. In this case, given the reassuring FHR once the fetal head is elevated off of the umbilical cord, spinal anesthesia is preferred.

A. Epidural anesthesia takes longer to reach a surgical level and is less often successful than spinal anesthesia. Epidural anesthesia is excellent for labor because continuous administration and titration for less neuromuscular block are possible.

C. In a true emergent cesarean delivery, if the anesthesiologist does not normally place many spinals, general anesthesia is commonly used. This patient may not be a good candidate for intubation, given her history of scleroderma. Ideally, the patient and her airway will have been evaluated by anesthesia at the time of her admission.

D. Occasionally, if anesthesia is unavailable, a cesarean section will be performed under local anesthesia with conscious sedation. This is certainly not an optimal way to perform surgery and, given the presence of an obstetric anesthesiologist in this case, is unnecessary here.

E. Pudendal anesthesia may be administered by an obstetrician prior to performing an operative vaginal delivery with vacuum or forceps but is not appropriate for cesarean delivery.

112. **B.** While variable decelerations and even prolonged decelerations are relatively common phenomena during labor, the sudden change of the fetal station from +2 to unpalpable and high is abnormal and highly concerning. In this setting of a patient undergoing a TOL after having had a prior cesarean delivery, the most likely diagnosis is a uterine rupture. Other common signs and symptoms associated with uterine rupture include a maternal "popping" sensation in the abdomen, extreme abdominal pain, palpation of fetal parts outside of the uterus, gush of vaginal bleeding, and maternal hypotension secondary to intra-abdominal bleeding. Even though the FHR returns to baseline, a rapid cesarean delivery is indicated.

A. Fetal scalp pH is likely to be relatively reassuring because there is still good FHR variability. Nevertheless, in this scenario, delivery should be facilitated.

C. Forceps cannot be used with a fetal head this high or a cervix that is not fully dilated.

D. Expectant management would be reasonable if uterine rupture did not appear to be the likely diagnosis. If the head were still at +2 station and there were no recurrences of the prolonged decelerations, the patient would ideally be completely dilated soon and could be delivered vaginally.

E. As with expectant management, if you did not suspect uterine rupture, you would restart the Pitocin about 20 to 30 minutes after the prolonged deceleration.

---

113. **C.** Wound infections are the most common complication of abdominal and pelvic surgery. They can consist of a simple cellulitis, a wound abscess, or a fasciitis; the last complication carries a relatively high rate of mortality. The next step in this patient's management is to further assess the wound. The simplest way to do so is at the bedside with local anesthesia. The incision should then be opened 1 to 2 cm to allow for exploration of the wound with a cotton swab. If the abscess is local and without much depth, the wound can be irrigated and packed with cotton gauze. Otherwise, consideration should be given to irrigation and debridement in the operating room.

A. The patient may require intravenous antibiotics depending on the extent of the wound infection. If she is admitted with a fasciitis, broad-spectrum antibiotics should be given. However, with a small wound abscess that is opened and packed, continuing the oral antibiotics for the accompanying cellulitis should be adequate.

B. If the infection is found to be quite extensive, or if the patient does not tolerate examination under local anesthesia, exploration in the OR may be necessary.

D. The wound should be irrigated, but not until it is explored.

E. A CT scan is sometimes used if a wound is closed and without obvious fluctuance but the cellulitis does not resolve after treatment. It can identify any enclosed areas of fluid or an intra-abdominal abscess.

---

114. **A.** This patient is likely intravascularly depleted. The first step in dealing with her oliguria is to give IV fluid. Patients who undergo abdominal surgery have large insensible losses. This patient also had approximately 4 L of ascites drained, is likely quite dry, and should receive aggressive hydration.

B. While this patient is likely down several liters of total fluid, a 2000-cc bolus is a bit aggressive in this situation and can cause pulmonary edema.

C. Salt-poor albumin (SPA) may be useful for this patient if several boluses of crystalloid fail to produce adequate urination. Patients with ovarian cancer often have low oncotic pressure secondary to low albumin, and boluses of colloid can improve intravascular volume at least temporarily.

D, E. Only if the patient normally takes a diuretic should one be given in the first 24 hours postoperatively for oliguria. While the patient is likely to show a response, the diuretic may leave her with even less intravascular fluid and may increase the risk of acute renal failure.

---

115. **B.** The average female patient has between 4 and 4.5 L of intravascular volume. Because this patient is larger than average, she may have as much as 5 L. Her blood loss during the case was approximately one third of her total blood volume. In addition, she was given a large fluid bolus to replace the volume. Now, 6 hours postoperatively, she has re-equilibrated most of the fluids. Appropriately, her hematocrit is approximately two thirds of her starting hematocrit.

A. In this stable patient with normal urine output, there is no reason to check serial hematocrits unless concern arises that she may have continued intra-abdominal bleeding.

C. In this stable patient, there is no reason to re-explore.

D. With a hematocrit of 28 and a stable patient, there is no need to transfuse blood. Occasionally, cancer patients or cardiac patients are transfused for hematocrits lower than 30 to prepare for chemotherapy or to maximize oxygen-carrying capacity.

E. There is no reason at this point to suspect a coagulopathy. If one was suspected, a better screening test is to check for fibrin split products such as the D-dimer.

116. **E.** Laparoscopic injuries to the bowel are rare and dangerous complications. The bowel can be injured during insertion of the Veress needle, insertion of the trochars, operative dissection using sharp instruments, and use of electrocautery—particularly unipolar electrocautery, as it can lead to arcing of sparks. Patients may present immediately or several days postoperatively with symptoms related to bowel perforation. In this patient with an acute abdomen and septic physiology, a bowel injury leading to a perforation is the most likely diagnosis. Of note, the free air seen on the upright abdominal film is concerning for ruptured viscus. However, it could also be secondary to remaining gas in the abdomen after surgery (as long as 7 days postoperatively).

A. Postoperative PID alone is unlikely in this patient, as it is usually seen in patients after the release of a hydrosalpinx that is filled with contaminated material. This patient's signs and symptoms indicate a systemic problem and are more consistent with the rupture of a viscus.

B. Endomyometritis should not create such widespread abdominal symptoms.

C. Appendicitis can present like this patient's signs and symptoms, but given the timing of the recent surgery, bowel injury is more likely. In either situation, consultation with general surgery and immediate abdominal exploration constitute the next step.

D. It is unlikely that ureteral injury would present with signs of infection and subsequent progression to sepsis.

117. **B.** Currently, first-line combination chemotherapy for patients with epithelial ovarian carcinoma consists of Taxol and carboplatin. Carboplatin has replaced cisplatin as the primary platinum-based alkylating agent because it is associated with fewer side effects.

A. CHOP is most commonly used to treat non-Hodgkin's lymphoma.

C. Melphalan was once a commonly used single agent to treat ovarian cancer. It is still used in patients who are less likely to survive combination therapy because it is well tolerated.

D. Etoposide and cisplatin are most commonly used to treat oat cell lung cancer.

E. CMF combination chemotherapy has been used to treat breast cancer, with and without tamoxifen.

118. **A.** With a ureteral transection above the pelvic brim, the best repair is to reapproximate the two ends over a stent. The stent helps to prevent stenosis from scarring during the healing process.

B. End-to-side reanastomosis is unusual in ureteral repair. It is used more commonly in bowel reanastomosis to prevent stenotic sites.

C. If a distal ureteral injury has occurred, reimplantation may be used over reanastomosis. In this case, the injury is too proximal to be reimplanted on the bladder.

D. End-to-side anastomosis may be used in ureteral repair when implanting the ureter into the contralateral ureter. This procedure is performed rarely in instances where the distal ureter has been resected and there is no way to bridge the distance between the ureter and the bladder.

E. When the ureter has been damaged to such an extent that there is not enough distance to implant into the bladder or contralateral ureter, a nephrostomy tube will be placed; it allows the kidney to continue functioning.

119. **B.** Heparin SQ dosed 5000 units BID or TID is most commonly used for DVT prophylaxis perioperatively. The original studies examined the TID dosing, which should be used in patients at highest risk (e.g., those with cancer). The BID dosing is commonly used in patients who are healthy and likely to mobilize quickly.

A. Coumadin has a slow onset and a long half-life. As a consequence, it is not used for perioperative prophylaxis.

C. LMW heparin such as Lovenox can be used for DVT prophylaxis, dosed at 40 units QD. However, because it has a longer half-life than unfractionated heparin, it is not usually used perioperatively.

D, E. See the explanations for A, B, and C.

120. **D.** The patient's infertility in this case is most likely related to her endometriosis. However, with good tubal patency on the left and some spillage on the right, it is impossible to say for certain that tubal factor is implicated. Patients with infertility secondary to endometriosis will have increased fertility with the fulguration of implants that are seemingly unrelated to the adnexa.

A. With pelvic adhesions, chronic PID is in the differential diagnosis. With an endometrioma, endometriosis is the most likely diagnosis.

B. While this is a possible etiology, it is unlikely to be the diagnosis in this patient as good tubal patency has been demonstrated on the left.

C. This patient with regular menses and documented ovulation does not have ovarian dysfunction.

E. This is incorrect on both accounts because there is both a clear etiology (i.e., endometriosis) and tubal patency.

121. **D.** Although most uterine perforations go unnoticed and are not associated with morbidity or mortality, recognition of a uterine perforation requires that one evaluate the patient for stability and intra-abdominal bleeding. The least invasive way to do so is to perform a pelvic US to look for blood or other fluid in the pelvis. In this case, because the hysteroscopy had not begun, minimal fluid should be present in the pelvis. Occasionally, if the patient is showing signs of cardiovascular instability, laparoscopy is performed to look for ongoing bleeding.

A. If a uterine perforation is recognized, it is unsafe to proceed with hysteroscopy because the fluid under pressure is likely to pass in large amounts into the abdomen through the perforation site. In addition, placement of the hysteroscope may further dilate or damage the perforation site.

B. Laparotomy is not needed, unless there is evidence of intra-abdominal bleeding from the perforation site. Laparoscopy could be performed if the concern for bleeding was quite high.

C. As noted in the explanation for A, the case should not be continued. Antibiotics are a reasonable addition to expectant management—usually broad-spectrum agents similar to those used for PID.

E. While most uterine perforations are not associated with long-term morbidity, it is still wise to admit the patient overnight for observation.

122. **D.** The patient will most likely require less insulin during labor, and certainly less after delivery, relative to her antepartum requirements. During pregnancy, placental products (e.g., human chorionic somatomammotropin and placental growth hormone) increase maternal resistance to insulin, thus increasing insulin requirements for patients with pregestational diabetes, and sometimes generating a new requirement for exogenous insulin in gestational diabetics. In the active intrapartum period, these requirements usually decrease secondary to the increased glucose metabolism by the uterus and other physiology of labor. It is important to carefully monitor the patient's blood sugars, as maintaining adequate control can be tough. Most pregestational diabetics will require a continuous insulin infusion to keep tight blood sugar control. After delivery, insulin requirements drop even further with the expulsion of the placenta and the loss of its counterregulatory products (which have short half-lives). For this reason, long-acting insulin is to be avoided near delivery, if possible, out of concern for inducing postpartum hypoglycemia. On discharge from the hospital, insulin is typically restarted at 66% to 100% of prepregnancy levels for overt diabetics. For gestational diabetics, insulin is usually withheld altogether, and a glucose tolerance test should be repeated at 6 weeks postpartum.

A, B, C, E. See the explanation for D.

123. | **E.** Preeclampsia is formally diagnosed by proteinuria (equal to or greater than 300 mg proteinuria/24 h, or persistent dipstick of 1+ or greater) and hypertension (BP greater than 140 mm Hg systolic or 90 mm Hg diastolic on two occasions at least 6 hours apart). Severe preeclampsia can be diagnosed based on increased thresholds for these values (protein level exceeding 5000 mg/24 h, or BP higher than 160/110), patient symptoms (e.g., severe headache, visual disturbances, RUQ pain), laboratory values (e.g., elevated liver transaminases, thrombocytopenia), or clinical assessment of oliguria or pulmonary edema. In this patient, RUQ pain and an elevated AST would make the diagnosis of severe preeclampsia.

A. This level of hypertension meets the criteria for mild, but not severe, preeclampsia.

B. This level of proteinuria meets the criteria for mild, but not severe, preeclampsia.

C. IUGR (fetal weight less than the 10th percentile), when combined with hypertension and proteinuria, is a particularly ominous sign for the fetus, reflecting uteroplacental insufficiency. In fact, some authors have proposed using IUGR as a criterion for severe preeclampsia; however, this choice remains debatable. In this case, the 13th percentile is of concern but does not merit immediate intervention if other fetal testing is reassuring.

D. Nondependent edema can be seen in both severe and mild preeclampsia. In addition, assessment of type or degree of edema is of limited utility in the diagnosis of preeclampsia, as it is rather nonspecific.

124. | **D.** This patient shows evidence of HELLP syndrome and immediate delivery is indicated. At 31 weeks, most obstetricians would manage this patient expectantly if her preeclampsia was mild, gaining additional time for fetal maturation until 35 to 36 weeks GA. With stable severe preeclampsia diagnosed only by elevated BPs or proteinuria, and with BPs controllable with medications, the most common choice is expectant management, at least until a full course of corticosteroids can be given. However, in the setting of HELLP syndrome, the risk to the mother (and the fetus) is too great to delay delivery. Corticosteroids should be continued, as evidence suggests that they may improve neonatal outcomes. It is also reasonable to attempt a trial of induction of labor to achieve a vaginal delivery. In any event, careful maternal and fetal monitoring is imperative, and cesarean delivery rates are certainly higher in these patients than in most patients undergoing a trial of induction of labor. Magnesium sulfate seizure prophylaxis should also be initiated.

A. See the explanation for D.

B. Cesarean delivery is generally reserved for obstetrical indications. In this patient, these indications may develop as nonreassuring fetal monitoring or rapidly changing maternal lab tests or other indications of maternal decompensation.

C. Tocolysis to gain time for steroid administration is a common obstetrical strategy in the setting of preterm labor, but would be of no benefit in the setting of HELLP syndrome.

E. This would be a reasonable strategy with the diagnosis of severe preeclampsia. In the setting of HELLP syndrome, magnesium sulfate should be initiated for seizure prophylaxis. However, expectant management is not appropriate.

125. **D.** Evidence that this outbreak is a primary infection, indicated by the absence of maternal anti-HSV IgG antibodies, elevates concern for disseminated disease in the neonate. Primary herpes infections carry a far greater risk of transmission to the fetus (as high as 50% if lesions are present at delivery) than do recurrent infections (less than 5%), and the risk of severe adverse neonatal outcomes is markedly increased. This higher risk is believed to be due to higher viral loads and the lack of protective transplacental maternal antibodies. A negative IgG titer indicates that the infection is primary, recent, and dangerous. Although infections may be limited to local lesions (e.g., sores on the skin and mouth), disseminated HSV (viral sepsis, pneumonia, encephalitis) is associated with a mortality rate greater than 50%. If this patient had not delivered in the ambulance, current guidelines would dictate cesarean delivery. Placental transmission of HSV is rare, and the vast majority of infection occurs through exposure to maternal lesions and viral shedding in the birth canal, which can be minimized with cesarean delivery.

A. The patient's prior outbreaks would suggest that this outbreak represents a secondary infection, which carries a much lower risk of transmission and disseminated disease.

B. The knowledge that this outbreak occurred in the second trimester does not help distinguish between primary and secondary infection. If this is indeed a primary infection, infection remote from delivery carries a lower risk of adverse neonatal outcome, as there is more time for protective maternal antibody formation.

C. A history of oral HSV-1 does not help distinguish between primary and secondary infection. If this is indeed a newly acquired HSV-2 infection, previous HSV-1 infection does mitigate the risk of adverse neonatal outcome; such an infection is known as a "nonprimary first infection." Cross-reactive HSV-1 antibodies, present in maternal serum, reduce the risk of transmission, and neonatal infections are generally less severe and shorter in duration.

E. Acyclovir beginning at 36 weeks GA has been shown to reduce positive culture rates and viral shedding. Although a benefit of reducing transmission rates has not been definitively demonstrated, acyclovir therapy would be reassuring, if anything, against the risk of disseminated disease.

126. **B.** Endomyometritis, commonly known as "childbed fever," is the most common cause of puerperal fever and involves infection of the decidua and superficial myometrium. Puerperal infection is defined as a temperature to 38.0°C (100.4°F) or higher for 2 of the first 10 days postpartum, exclusive of the first 24 hours. The single greatest risk factor for puerperal infection is the route of delivery, with cesarean delivery conferring a higher risk. Additional risk factors for postpartum uterine infection include chorioamnionitis, multiple cervical exams, prolonged rupture of membranes, internal fetal monitoring, and lower socioeconomic status.

A. Infection of a vaginal hematoma presents with exquisite pain in the vaginal area and is less commonly associated with a high fever and rigors. Vaginal hematomas are detected by physical exam and the presence of a firm, tender mass. Large vaginal hematomas require drainage.

C. Deep vein thrombosis (DVT) most commonly occurs in the lower extremities and is associated with puerperal temperature elevations. Classic puerperal deep vein thrombophlebitis, also known as phlegmasia alba dolens (milk leg), has a rapid onset and is associated with a painful and edematous leg and thigh. Doppler studies should be ordered when a lower-extremity DVT is of concern. Thrombophlebitis of the pelvic venous plexuses also occurs and should be considered if fever spikes continue despite adequate antibiotic therapy and exclusion of an abscess.

D. Pyelonephritis can present with fever and rigors in the postpartum period; unilateral lower back pain is often a concomitant complaint. Costovertebral angle tenderness on physical exam also increases one's suspicion for pyelonephritis. A urine analysis with microscopy should be performed as well as culture with sensitivities. Pregnant women are at increased risk for pyelonephritis secondary to mass compression of the ureters and bladder. Bladder catheterization is a risk factor for urinary tract infections.

E. Pneumonia also can present with a fever and rigors in the postpartum period, but a cough is often present with this diagnosis. In the absence of intubation, as for an emergent cesarean delivery, postpartum pneumonia is rather uncommon. Intubation increases one's risk for aspiration pneumonia, most commonly in the right lower lobe. Unilobar rales are often present on physical exam. A chest radiograph should be ordered if pneumonia is under serious consideration. A major cause of pneumonia in pregnancy is preceding pyelonephritis.

127. **B.** The first steps in evaluation of a patient with a fever should be a review of the patient's course, a brief patient interview, and a physical exam. In this patient, a bimanual exam should be performed as part of the physical exam. The external perineum and vagina should be inspected for hematoma formation, episiotomy infection/dehiscence, and evidence of necrotizing fasciitis. The cervix should be assessed for cervical motion tenderness and masses concerning for a cervical hematoma. The uterine body and parametria should be assessed for tenderness, size, and masses. Return of malodorous lochia or clot should be noted. The work-up of a puerperal fever also includes a urinalysis and, depending on the clinical scenario, a CBC and blood cultures.

A. Chest X-ray should be ordered only if there is a heightened clinical suspicion of a respiratory process, such as pneumonia or pulmonary edema.

C. A pelvic US may be useful if a bimanual exam raises concern for an infected hematometrium (blood in the uterus) or other pelvic mass. A pelvic US is not diagnostic for endomyometritis.

D. Before ordering a lower-extremity Doppler, one should first perform a physical exam. Typical findings with a lower-extremity DVT include asymmetric edema (if asymmetry is unclear, one should measure the circumference of each calf with a measuring tape), tenderness to palpation of the calf, presence of a palpable cord in the lower extremity, erythema, and a positive Homan's sign (calf pain elicited by dorsiflexion of the foot). Of note, Homan's sign is present in 50% of cases where a DVT is confirmed as well as 50% of cases where a DVT is excluded. Although its clinical utility is as good as flipping a coin, it is nonetheless a favored diagnostic criterion on standardized exams.

E. Sputum culture is rarely helpful in any clinical setting, with the exceptions being evaluation of tuberculosis and ventilated patients.

128. **B.** *E. coli* is a gram-negative rod that grows under aerobic conditions and is a common cause of pelvic infections.

A. *S. epidermidis* is a skin flora that is not a common cause of pelvic infection.

C, D, E. In addition to *E. coli*, these are common pathogens of puerperal pelvic infections. The causal factor is that they are bacteria that normally reside in the bowel and commonly colonize the perineum, vagina, and cervix. Although routinely sterile, the uterus can become colonized by ascending pathogens after rupture of the amniotic membranes. Common pathogens include: Group A, B, and D *Streptococcus*, *Enterococcus* species, gram-negatives (*E. coli* and *Klebsiella*), *Staphylococcus aureus*, *Peptostreptococcus*, *Bacteroides fragilis*, *Clostridium* spp., *Chlamydia trachomatis*, and *Neisseria gonorrheae*. However, *Enterococcus* is a gram-positive coccus, *B. fragilis* is an anaerobic organism, and *C. trachomatis* is an intracellular organism that is difficult to culture and most commonly detected by DNA tests.

129. **C.** Colostrum is the initial yellow liquid produced by the breast as a result of pregnancy. Colostrum production occurs during the first 5 postpartum days and then gradually converts to mature milk production over the course of approximately 4 weeks. Compared to mature milk, colostrum has more protein. It also carries immunoglobulin A, which is thought to confer early protection again enteric pathogens to the breastfed neonate.

A. Colostrum contains less fat than mature milk.

B. Colostrum contains more minerals than mature milk.

D. Colostrum has less sugar than mature milk.

E. See the explanations for A, B, C, and D.

130. **C.** Oxytocin, released from the posterior pituitary, is responsible for the milk "let-down" reflex. This reflex mechanism may be provoked by nipple stimulation, such as suckling, or the cry of an infant. Stress and fright may inhibit the reflex.

A. Estrogen plays a role in breast maturation but does not directly cause milk ejection.

B. Prolactin, released by the anterior pituitary gland, stimulates milk production, not milk "let-down."

D. Placental lactogen does not cause milk "let-down" and is produced only by the placenta; thus, after the third stage of labor, it is no longer produced.

E. There is no hormone called stimulactogen.

131. **B.** Infants who are breastfed have a lower incidence of ear infections as compared to formula-fed infants. This difference is attributed in part to the passive maternal antibodies contained in breast milk, which provide the infant with passive immunity to many neonatal and infantile infections.

A. Breastfed infants have fewer allergies, both as infants and subsequently as adults, than do formula-fed infants.

C. Women who breastfeed their infants lose their "pregnancy weight" faster than women who bottle-feed their babies. Breastfeeding consumes, on average, 500 kilocalories per day, while pregnancy requires only an additional 300 kilocalories per day.

D. Typically, infants who are fed formula gain weight more rapidly and tend to continue to be heavier as compared to infants who are fed breast milk. Some speculate that the increased weight (and percentage of body fat) of formula-fed infants sets their metabolism such that they are more prone to becoming obese as adults.

E. It has been reported that breastfed infants gain unique protection from Crohn's disease, ulcerative colitis, certain lymphomas, diabetes, pneumonia, and meningitis. However, no studies to date suggest lower rates of autism in breastfed infants.

132. **D.** Prolonged crowning of the fetal head followed by the "turtle" sign (incomplete delivery of the fetal head followed by retraction into the vagina after pushing) is suggestive of shoulder dystocia. Gestational diabetes and prolonged second stage are risk factors. Other risk factors include fetal macrosomia, previous dystocia, maternal obesity, and post-dates delivery. A series of maneuvers exist for delivering an infant with shoulder dystocia, including the following: (1) McRoberts maneuver (Figure 132), a sharp ventral rotation of both maternal hips bringing the pelvic inlet and outlet into a more vertical alignment, and facilitating delivery of the fetal shoulders; (2) suprapubic pressure, to dislodge the anterior shoulder from behind the pubic symphysis; (3) Rubin maneuver; (4) Wood's corkscrew maneuver; and (5) delivery of the posterior arm/shoulder. These maneuvers may be repeated if they prove unsuccessful the first time. If the infant is still undelivered, episiotomy or fracturing the fetal clavicle may be indicated for delivery.

A. Gentle downward traction alone is often insufficient initial management of shoulder dystocia. Strong, jerking, downward traction of the head is never appropriate, as it can lead to fetal injury.

B, C. Vacuum-assisted and forceps-assisted deliveries are contraindicated when shoulder dystocia is suspected, as both are associated with a slightly increased rate of shoulder dystocia. In this patient, because the head has already delivered, neither of these devices offers any benefit.

E. Uterine fundal pressure is contraindicated in the event of shoulder dystocia, as it will lead to further impaction of the shoulder behind the pubic symphysis.

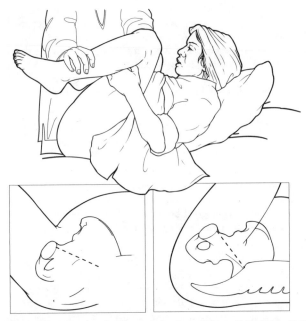

Figure 132 • Reproduced with permission from Callahan T. Blueprints Obstetrics & Gynecology. 3rd ed. Blackwell, 2004: Fig. 6-7, p. 70.

133. **B.** The principal benefit of prolonging pregnancy for an additional 48 hours is that it allows treatment with steroids. Betamethasone, a glucocorticoid, has been shown to decrease the incidence of respiratory distress syndrome and other complications from preterm delivery.

A. No evidence exists that treatment of preterm labor with antibiotics prolongs pregnancy. Strong evidence, however, indicates that the use of antibiotics in PPROM leads to a longer latency period prior to the onset of labor.

C. Although magnesium sulfate has been shown to stop contractions in small placebo-controlled trials, it has not been shown to change the GA at delivery. Many of the tocolytics used have been shown to make a difference only by prolonging gestation for 48 hours.

D. Intravenous magnesium sulfate is also used in pregnant patients with preeclampsia to decrease the risk of seizures. This patient does not have preeclampsia, so it would not be used for this reason.

E. See the explanation for B.

134. **B.** Sudden onset of profuse, painless vaginal bleeding is indicative of placenta previa. Risk factors for placenta previa include history of prior placenta previa or cesarean section, multiparity, multiple gestation, erythroblastosis, smoking, and increasing maternal age. As most patients who receive prenatal care in the United States undergo a second trimester US, placenta previa is usually diagnosed prior to the classic presentation that this woman has experienced.

A. The classic presentation of placental abruption is vaginal bleeding associated with severe abdominal pain, typically occurring in the third trimester. Physical exam often reveals a firm, tender uterus. Small, frequent uterine contractions are usually seen on tocometry. Additionally, fetal monitoring may be nonreassuring secondary to uteroplacental insufficiency. Risk factors for placental abruption include history of prior placental abruption, hypertension, substance use, trauma, and multiple gestation.

C. Cervical cancer may cause vaginal bleeding in its advanced stages. The classic presentation of advanced cervical cancer is postcoital bleeding. Other signs and symptoms that may accompany cervical cancer include abnormal vaginal bleeding, watery discharge, pelvic pain or pressure, and rectal or urinary symptoms. On speculum exam, an exophytic lesion on the cervix may be visible. Given that women are routinely screened prenatally via Pap smears and that cervical cancer is generally a slowly progressing cancer, occurrence of advanced-stage cervical cancer during pregnancy is rare.

D. While labor can cause some vaginal bleeding, it is rarely a large amount and more often is described as "bloody show," or bloody mucus. Preterm labor is defined as uterine contractions that cause a cervical change prior to 37 weeks GA. This patient is not experiencing contractions.

E. Hemorrhoids do lead to rectal bleeding that can be confused with vaginal bleeding antepartum. However, the bleeding is generally greatest at the end of pregnancy, is associated with bowel movements, and rarely would be heavy enough to soak a towel.

135. **C.** Many changes in the pulmonary, renal, and hematologic systems occur during pregnancy. In this scenario, the patient has many complaints but the most concerning lab result is her hypercarbia, indicating pulmonary compromise. In pregnancy, the tidal volume increases by approximately 40% while the respiratory rate remains unchanged, leading to an increase in the minute ventilation. An increase in the minute ventilation produces increases in the alveolar and arterial O_2 levels and decreases in the alveolar and arterial CO_2 levels (normal $PaCO_2$ in pregnancy is 30 mm Hg). This patient is retaining CO_2, which is abnormal and concerning.

A. The glomerular filtration rate increases by approximately 50% in pregnancy, leading to a lower BUN and creatinine levels. Additionally, the renin-angiotensin system creates elevated levels of aldosterone, which keeps serum sodium levels normal.

B. The WBC count increases in pregnancy, with the upper limit of normal being 16. In fact, the WBC count is often 20 million/mL during labor.

D. Pregnancy-related changes in hemoglobin and hematocrit occur as the plasma volume increases by 50% but the RBC volume increases by 25%, leading to a lower hematocrit during pregnancy.

E. Many pregnant women experience an iron-deficiency anemia secondary to the increase in RBC mass.

136. **D.** This patient has recurrent cervical incompetence and may have benefited from a cervical cerclage at an earlier GA (12 to 14 weeks). However, with her history of past losses and the current cervical exam, it is reasonable to offer a cerclage now. A cerclage is a permanent suture placed at the cervical–vaginal junction (McDonald) or at the internal os (Shirodkar) to close the cervix. The complications from its placement can be disastrous, including infection and PPROM. Typical management of previable cervical incompetence is cerclage placement (if cervical dilation and effacement are not too great), expectant management, or elective termination.

A. In the setting of incompetent cervix with the membranes pushing down through the cervix (prolapsing membranes), strict bedrest is a less interventional modality that may be offered. Betamethasone for fetal lung maturity would not be utilized until the fetus reached viability (24 weeks GA).

B. Antibiotics are not efficacious in the management of cervical incompetence. They are used commonly in the setting of PPROM to increase the time period from ROM to the onset of labor (latency).

C. As noted in the explanation for A, bedrest in the Trendelenburg position may be employed in the setting of advanced cervical dilation with prolapsing membranes. In theory, this positioning with the maternal head below the pelvis allows gravity to facilitate the membranes moving back up the cervix, thereby reducing the forces on the cervix. However, a cerclage is more likely to be beneficial to this patient.

E. Tocolytics are administered when a patient has uterine contractions, but they are rarely used in the previable fetus.

137. **B.** Asthma and glaucoma are contraindications for the use of prostaglandins. Obstetric contraindications include uterine contractions as frequent as every 5 minutes and prior cesarean delivery or other uterine scar. Relative contraindications include oligohydramnios (AFI less than 5 cm at term) and IUGR, but prostaglandins can still be used in these settings if a negative contraction stress test with oxytocin precedes their use.

A, C, D, E. See the explanation for B. Hypertension (including the hypertension of preeclampsia) is a contraindication to the use of Methergine (methylergonovine), a medicine employed to treat uterine atony as an etiology for postpartum hemorrhage. However, prostaglandins may be used in the setting of hypertension.

138. **A.** Fetal scalp sampling for pH is rarely used, but it is a direct measure to assess possible fetal acidemia. The clinical setting in this case is one in which fetal scalp sampling is useful. There is nothing reassuring about the FHR tracing and with a failed fetal scalp stimulation, the next step is often immediate delivery. However, in a multiparous patient who may be an hour or so from delivery, a reassuring fetal scalp sample buys enough time to expectantly manage the patient. A fetal scalp sample that is greater than 7.25 is reassuring, so expectant management is appropriate.

B, C. A fetal scalp pH of less than 7.20 is nonreassuring, and in such a case the fetus should be delivered via cesarean section or assisted vaginal delivery. At a pH of 7.10, delivering the fetus rather than taking the time to resample is the appropriate action. Similarly, a pH of 7.15 also merits delivery rather than expectant management.

D. A scalp pH of 7.55 should alert the practitioner to contamination, possibly with amniotic fluid, and should lead to resampling rather than moving immediately to delivery.

E. When the scalp pH is between 7.20 and 7.25, the fetus is slightly below normal and the scalp pH should be resampled within a short period of time (less than 30 minutes) if the indication for assessing fetal pH persists. A cesarean section for a pH of 7.22 is unnecessary.

139. **C.** The most likely cause of the FHR deceleration is a tetanic contraction (contraction lasting more than 2 minutes). The long contraction squeezes venous blood out of the uterus and limits arterial perfusion. The placental unit is subsequently affected, the fetus becomes hypoxic, and the heart rate falls for a prolonged period of time—$4\frac{1}{2}$ minutes in this case. Tetanic contraction can be diagnosed by palpation of a firm, contracting uterus that does not relent. The length of the contraction can also be seen in the tocometer portion of the FHT shown (see Figure 139).

A. Cord compression is a possible cause of prolonged decelerations. In this setting, given the prolonged uterine contraction and no resolution secondary to patient manipulation, the tetanic contraction is the more likely etiology.

B. Placenta previa would present in the early stages of labor with profuse vaginal bleeding. Patients with placenta previa must have a cesarean delivery for maternal and fetal safety.

D. Cord prolapse can result in prolonged deceleration or bradycardia but is exceedingly uncommon when the fetal vertex is engaged. Furthermore, a cord prolapse is usually noted on vaginal exam, with the cord looping down past the fetal head and into the vagina.

E. A precipitous delivery may rarely be associated with a prolonged deceleration due to head or cord compression. However, in this instance, the fetus is at –1 station.

140. **C.** Discontinuation of the Pitocin infusion with administration of 0.25 mg terbutaline subcutaneously will likely resolve the prolonged uterine contraction, allowing for perfusion of the placental unit. Tetanic uterine contraction or hypertonus is diagnosed by palpating the contracted uterus, verifying the prolonged contraction of the external monitor, or IUPC.

A. If the FHT does not recover within a few moments or the preceding measures do not resolve the tetanic contraction, an emergent cesarean section must be performed.

B. The cervical exam confirming that the vertex is at –1 station eliminates forceps-assisted vaginal delivery as an option.

D. In the setting of cord prolapse, elevation of the fetal vertex is important to keep the umbilical cord from being occluded. In this setting, however, it has no utility.

E. Scalp pH sampling is helpful when long-term metabolic changes are expected (i.e., after 30 minutes of an abnormal FHT).

141. **B.** When a patient's cervical exam remains unchanged for 2 hours despite adequate forces (180 to 200 Montevideo units during contractions over 10 minutes), the diagnosis of active-phase arrest is made. It is an indication for cesarean section.

A. The fetal heart tracing (FHT) overall is reassuring and not an indication for cesarean section.

C. This patient is still in the active part of the first stage of labor. The second stage begins with complete cervical dilation.

D. The uterine forces are adequate by the 200 Montevideo unit convention.

E. There is no need to continue labor based on the adequacy of uterine contractions, as the patient's cervix is unlikely to change.

142. **A.** A normal magnesium level in healthy individuals ranges from 1.5 to 3 mg/dL. At 4 to 7 mg/dL, the level is therapeutic for seizure prevention. One will begin to see EKG changes from 5 to 10 mg/dL, loss of the deep tendon reflexes at 8 to 12 mg/dL, warmth and flushing at 9 to 12 mg/dL, and somnolence and slurred speech at 10 to 12 mg/dL. However, muscle weakness/paralysis or respiratory difficulty does not manifest itself until 15 to 17 mg/dL. Cardiac arrest is also a real danger of magnesium overdose, although it does not occur until levels approach 25 to 30 mg/dL or higher.

B, D. See the explanation for A.

C. Increased magnesium levels decrease the rate of seizures.

E. While diplopia and blurry vision are common side effects from elevated magnesium levels, blindness is not associated with magnesium use and should be attributed to the underlying preeclampsia.

143. **A.** Metastasis to the placenta and, more rarely, to the fetus have been reported. Although extremely uncommon, the greatest risk for metastasis to either mother or baby is seen with melanoma, leukemia, lymphoma, and breast cancer.

B. Chemotherapeutic agents are contraindicated in the first trimester, during organogenesis, because they may be teratogenic and mutagenic. They are relatively safe later in pregnancy.

C. Breast cancer diagnosed during pregnancy is no different than that diagnosed in the nonpregnant state, but the diagnosis is usually delayed during pregnancy due to physiologic changes in the breast, resulting in a more advanced stage and poorer survival rate at diagnosis.

D. Radiation therapy is contraindicated during pregnancy. It may cause spontaneous abortion, growth restriction, and mental retardation.

E. Termination of pregnancy may be needed to proceed with treatment such as radiation therapy, but it does not change the course of the malignancy.

144. | **C.** Embryonal carcinomas may produce hCG, AFP, and CA-125.

A. Choriocarcinoma is a germ cell tumor, also a form of gestational trophoblastic disease, which secretes hCG, not AFP.

B. Dysgerminoma, a germ cell tumor of the ovary affecting predominantly girls and young women, is remarkable for its secretion of LDH as a tumor marker. Germ cell tumors of the ovary arise from totipotential cells. Patients commonly present with a rapidly enlarging adnexal mass and abdominal pain. Functioning germ cell tumors of other types may produce tumor markers including AFP, hCG, and CA-125.

D. Endodermal sinus tumors may produce AFP.

E. Immature teratomas, or immature dermoid cysts, may produce CA-125.

145. | **B.** This image shows a submucosal fibroid. Menorrhagia is a common symptom of fibroids, particularly submucosal fibroids, which can distort their overlying endometrium and erode into the endometrial cavity.

A. This image does not show cervical cancer, which is better characterized on CT scan (although CT scan is not a formal part of the staging process). While cervical cancer lesions can bleed, they rarely lead to acute blood loss and anemia of this magnitude.

C. This image does not show an adnexal mass. Additionally, ovarian cancer does not typically lead to menorrhagia. If the mass secretes such large amounts of estrogen that the endometrium is stimulated, vaginal bleeding can occur, but is unlikely to be severe.

D. Endometrial polyps are difficult to diagnose on US unless fluid is instilled into the uterine cavity (known as a water or saline US). They are best identified on hysteroscopy or endometrial biopsy. Typically, they cause metrorrhagia rather than severe menorrhagia.

E. This image does not show a TOA. Also, TOAs are not associated with menorrhagia.

146. | **D.** Hysteroscopic resection is a minimally invasive treatment option for removal of lesions in the endometrial cavity such as fibroids and endometrial polyps.

A. In thermal balloon ablation, the endometrial lining is destroyed by heat in an effort to treat dysfunctional uterine bleeding once malignancy has been ruled out. It is not an appropriate treatment option for submucosal fibroids.

B, C. LEEP is an office procedure utilized to excise cervical abnormalities such as LSIL and HSIL. Similarly to LEEP, cone biopsies are performed in the setting of cervical rather than intrauterine abnormalities.

E. While hysterectomy is used in the treatment of fibroids, it is usually implemented after more conservative options such as medical therapy have failed. Of note, hysteroscopic resection is appropriate only for fibroids accessible via the endometrial cavity (i.e., submucosal fibroids). If hysterectomy were to be performed, one must take into account the patient's age and determine whether it would be appropriate to perform a bilateral salpingo-oophorectomy at the same time. In this patient who is likely quite remote from menopause (average age of menopause is 50 years), excision of the ovaries would likely be inadvisable given the premature surgical menopause that would result.

147. **C.** Postoperative sources of fever include atelectasis, urinary tract infection, deep vein thrombosis, medications, and infection of the wound, lungs, or abdomen. With a relatively low-grade temperature (less than 101°F) and decreased breath sounds, the most likely diagnosis is atelectasis. Appropriate management involves encouragement of incentive spirometry and ambulation, both of which will help re-expand the lungs. The patient's temperatures should be observed, as true infections will continue to cause fevers.

A. Without complaints of dysuria or hematuria and without an indwelling catheter, the likelihood of urinary tract infection is low. However, this possibility could easily be investigated with a urinalysis and urine culture.

B. There is no wound erythema or drainage, making a wound cellulitis or infection unlikely.

D. While this patient is at increased risk of thromboembolic events such as DVT due to her obesity and immobility postoperatively, her exam does not reveal any palpable cords, nor does she complain of difficulty ambulating.

E. Postoperative infections can arise from the wound, lungs, urine, and (rarely) retained foreign bodies such as laparotomy sponges. If a patient mounts significant temperatures and exam is suggestive of a pulmonary or urinary tract etiology, appropriate studies should be obtained. In particular, if a patient has signs and symptoms concerning for a pulmonary embolus (e.g., tachycardia, shortness of breath, decreased oxygen saturation), a spiral CT scan should be obtained. If there is concern for sepsis, blood cultures can be sent. Additionally, the patient can be symptomatically treated with acetaminophen while awaiting diagnostic evaluation. This patient's exam is suggestive of atelectasis, so a full infection work-up is not necessary at this time.

148. **C.** This patient's exam is concerning for continued blood loss with a likely intra-abdominal source. The first step would be to check a stat hemoglobin/hematocrit to see whether it is consistent with her reported EBL and subsequent intravenous fluid hydration. Intravenous fluids should be continued, and a fluid bolus should be administered to see whether urine output increases in response, which would be suggestive of decreased intravascular volume. In the setting of large bloody drainage from the wound, decreased urine output, and vital signs concerning for decreased intravascular volume, if the blood count is lower than expected, consideration should be given to taking the patient back to the operating room for repeat exploratory laparotomy. Another diagnostic option that was not an answer choice is a bedside US to look for large amounts of intra-abdominal fluid suggestive of intra-abdominal bleeding.

A. While abdominal X-ray might show findings suggestive of increased abdominal fluid concerning for continued blood loss, it is not the best method to explore this possibility.

B. Occasionally, decreased urine output is falsely demonstrated secondary to a clogged or kinked Foley catheter. In this setting, using a syringe to inject saline into the bladder to unclog or kink the catheter ("flushing the Foley") is usually reasonable. Removing the catheter would be unwise, as you are using urine output as a crude assessment of renal perfusion.

D. See the explanation for C.

E. If you do remove the patient's staples so soon postoperatively, her wound will separate. This may be part of an exploratory laparotomy, but it would not be the initial step in assessment.

149. | **B.** This patient has a postoperative ileus, as evidenced by her symptom of nausea, signs of vomiting, abdominal distention, and the KUB image with air–fluid levels. Such a patient should remain NPO until she begins to pass flatus. While NPO, she must also receive IV hydration. In the case of a prolonged ileus, total parenteral nutrition (TPN) is used in addition to hydration. Of note, risk factors for ileus in this patient include extensive bowel manipulation during surgery, minimal postoperative mobility, and liberal use of narcotics.

A. In this patient with a postoperative ileus, she should be made NPO, rather than advancing her diet.

C. If such a patient has evidence for acute hemorrhage or a ruptured or torsed viscus, then exploratory laparotomy may be necessary. Hemorrhage would be suspected in the case of unstable vital signs or decreased urine output. Bowel injury will usually lead to an acute abdomen with peritoneal signs, which are not seen in this patient.

D. While the patient should be made NPO, nasogastric decompression of the ileus is usually unnecessary in gynecologic surgery unless aggressive manipulation of the bowel occurs during the procedure. Although the use of a nasogastric tube is not wrong, it certainly is less important than the IV hydration.

E. In the case of an ileus, oral bowel stimulants such as milk of magnesia (MOM) or GoLYTELY are likely to exacerbate the problem. By stimulating the bowel proximal to the ileus, greater distention and abdominal pain will be caused. Some physicians will use suppository agents such as Dulcolax or even enemas to stimulate the distal bowel in an attempt to relieve some of the symptoms. However, these methods have not been studied in prospective trials and little evidence supports their use in the case of an ileus.

150. | **B.** The major types of sex-cord stromal tumors include granulosa-theca and Sertoli-Leydig cell tumors and gonadoblastomas.

A. Epithelial cell tumors (rather than germ cell tumors) are the most common and give rise to benign and malignant tumors. Major categories of epithelial tumors include serous and mucinous tumors, endometrioid clear cell tumors, undifferentiated carcinomas, and Brenner tumors.

C, D. While epithelial cell tumors can affect women at any age, they occur most frequently among women in their late fifties. Germ cell tumors generally affect girls and women ages 0 to 25 years. Like all tumors, however, they may be seen at any age.

E. Mucinous and endometrioid tumors are considered epithelial cell neoplasms. Germ cell tumors include teratomas, dysgerminomas, endodermal sinus tumors, and choriocarcinomas. Ovarian neoplasms are classified by the cell type of origin: surface epithelial, germ, and sex-cord stromal cells.

Questions

Setting 4: Emergency Department

Generally, patients encountered here are seeking urgent care; most are not known to you. A full range of social services is available, including rape crisis intervention, family support, child protective services, domestic violence support, psychiatric services, and security assistance backed up by local police. Complete laboratory and radiology services are available.

151. A 32-year-old G_2P_1 woman at 33 1/7 weeks GA presents to the ED complaining of severe, nonradiating, right-sided abdominal pain that worsens with movement. She has not eaten since last night due to recurrent nausea and vomiting that started this morning, and her last bowel movement was yesterday. She denies travel, sick contacts, or food poisoning. The pregnancy has been uncomplicated. Physical exam is significant for a temperature of 101.0°F, abdominal guarding, rebound, and tenderness to palpation over the right middle abdomen. The patient's cervix is closed and not effaced on vaginal exam. Contractions are not detectable on tocometer, and fetal heart tracing is reassuring. Laboratory studies reveal a WBC count of 20,000 with a left shift. Urinalysis reveals only mild ketones. What is the appropriate diagnosis and treatment for this patient?

A. Diverticulosis—stool softeners
B. Preterm labor—tocolysis
C. Nephrolithiasis—hydration and pain control
D. Placental abruption—immediate delivery
E. Appendicitis—exploratory laparotomy

152. A 19-year-old G_1P_0 woman at 39 2/7 weeks GA presents complaining of constant epigastric pain and severe nausea and vomiting that started this afternoon. She has been receiving regular prenatal care and reports that the pregnancy has been uncomplicated. On further questioning, she states that she has also had a headache all day, but no visual disturbances. Physical exam is significant for normal temperature and BP, tenderness to palpation in the right upper quadrant of the abdomen, hyperreflexia, and 2+ lower-extremity edema as well as mild hand and facial edema. Vaginal exam reveals a cervix that is 2 cm dilated and 90% effaced. Tocometer reveals occasional contractions, and fetal heart tracing is reassuring. Urine dip reveals 1+ proteinuria. What is the most important next step in diagnosis and treatment of this patient?

A. IV fluids and pain control
B. Check preeclamptic labs, initiate magnesium prophylaxis, and move toward delivery
C. Tocolysis
D. Right upper quadrant US and pain control
E. Urgent cesarean section

153. A 23-year-old nonpregnant woman presents to the ED with sudden-onset, severe left-sided abdominal pain that is now mildly improved. She reports moderate pelvic discomfort over the past week, but denies fever, vomiting, vaginal discharge or bleeding, or bowel or bladder abnormalities. Her LMP was normal and occurred 2 weeks ago. She is sexually active, uses condoms, and has never had an STD. On physical exam, she has normal vital signs, is moderately tender to palpation in the left lower quadrant, has no cervical motion tenderness, and has no palpable adnexal or uterine masses. A urine pregnancy test is negative, and CBC shows a normal white count and hematocrit of 39. US is performed (Figure 153). What is the appropriate next step in this patient's management?

A. Diagnostic laparoscopy
B. IV antibiotics
C. Abdominal/pelvic CT scan
D. Pain relief and discharge home with precautions and outpatient follow-up
E. D&C

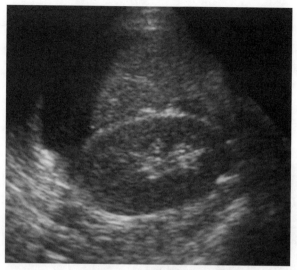

Figure 153 · Image provided by Departments of Radiology and Obstetrics & Gynecology, University of California, San Francisco.

The next two questions (items 154 and 155) correspond to the following vignette.

A 17-year-old nonpregnant woman presents to the ED complaining of suprapubic pain of 3 days duration. She has decreased her fluid intake because she is urinating so frequently, which worsens the pain and also causes a burning sensation. She denies fever, discharge, or GI symptoms. She just became sexually active and recently started using birth control pills. On physical exam, she is afebrile and has moderate tenderness to palpation in the suprapubic region. Bimanual exam reproduces the suprapubic discomfort, but is otherwise within normal limits.

154. Which of the following combination of urinalysis abnormalities is most consistent with her symptoms and likely diagnosis?

 A. WBCs, lipids
 B. WBCs, calcium deposits
 C. RBCs, renal epithelium
 D. Nitrites, WBCs, renal epithelium
 E. Nitrites, WBCs, leukocyte esterase, RBCs

155. Which of the following measures is appropriate management of this patient?

 A. Decrease fluid intake
 B. Foley catheter
 C. Urine culture and sensitivity
 D. IV antibiotics
 E. Low protein diet

End of set

156. A 17-year-old G_0 woman with a history of dysmenorrhea and menorrhagia presents to the ED complaining of gradual-onset lower abdominal pain and heavy vaginal bleeding that has soaked five pads over the past 12 hours. The patient is not sexually active. Her vital signs are stable, and she is afebrile. Physical exam reveals normal bowel sounds and mild lower abdominal tenderness to palpation, but no peritoneal signs or palpable masses. On pelvic exam, you note a small amount of blood in the vaginal vault, but no evidence of active bleeding, and no cervical motion tenderness or adnexal masses. Pelvic US is performed (Figure 156). The patient's hematocrit is 31. In addition to starting iron supplementation, which of the following measures would be appropriate management of this patient?

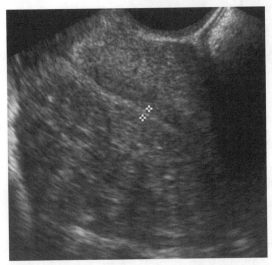

Figure 156 • Image provided by Departments of Radiology and Obstetrics & Gynecology, University of California, San Francisco.

    A. D&C
    B. Cyclic OCPs
    C. Gonadotropin-releasing hormone (GnRH) therapy
    D. Endometrial ablation
    E. Progestin trial (Depo-Provera)

157. A 47-year-old G_3P_3 woman with a history of menorrhagia and fibroids presents to the ED with a 5-day history of severe vaginal bleeding and complaining of weakness and dyspnea on exertion. Physical exam reveals a pale woman with tachycardia and orthostatic hypotension. Speculum exam is significant for a small amount of bleeding from the cervical os, and bimanual exam reveals an 8-week-sized uterus. The patient's hematocrit is 16.1. You obtain an US (Figure 157). What is the next step in treatment?

    A. Administer depot Lupron
    B. Blood transfusion
    C. Observation
    D. Hysterectomy
    E. Endometrial ablation

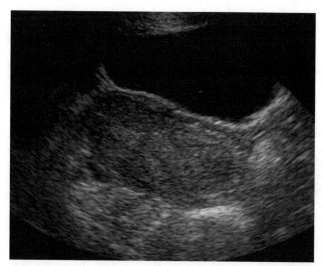

Figure 157 · Image provided by Departments of Radiology and Obstetrics & Gynecology, University of California, San Francisco.

158. A 32-year-old G_2P_1 at 31 5/7 weeks GA presents with painless vaginal bleeding that started today while she was walking. She reports soaking a hand towel with bright red blood, but denies leakage of fluid, contractions, trauma, intercourse, history of abnormal Pap smears, hematuria, hemorrhoids, or bleeding per rectum. On further questioning, she recalls being told at her 18-week US that her placenta was "over" her cervix, but failed to keep subsequent follow-up US appointments. Fetal heart tones are reassuring, and tocometer shows rare uterine contractions. The patient is hemodynamically stable and no longer having vaginal bleeding. Bedside abdominal US confirms complete placenta previa. What is the most appropriate next step in treatment?

A. Immediate delivery
B. Blood transfusion
C. Amniocentesis for fetal lung maturity
D. Administration of IV estrogen
E. Observation and administration of corticosteroids

159. A 22-year-old nonpregnant woman presents to the ED with bilateral groin pain and fever for several days. She is sexually active with two partners and uses the birth control patch for contraception. Her past gynecologic history is significant for hospitalization at age 19 for PID and treatment of chlamydia last year. On exam, she has enlarged inguinal lymph nodes bilaterally, but her abdomen is benign, and she does not have cervical motion tenderness or vaginal discharge. Which of the following statements is true regarding lymphogranuloma venereum (LGV)?

A. It is caused by the L serotypes of *Chlamydia trachomatis*
B. It typically starts out with a painful lesion in the genital region
C. Treatment involves a 3-week course of doxycycline and surgical exploration of lymph nodes
D. Involvement is usually limited to the lymph nodes
E. It is not sexually transmitted

160. A 30-year-old G_1P_1 comes to the ED complaining of progressive difficulty walking over the past day due to vaginal pain. She was discharged from the hospital the previous day after undergoing precipitous vaginal delivery of a 9 lb infant during which she sustained a second-degree vaginal laceration that was repaired. Physical exam is significant for mild tachycardia; neurologic exam is normal. The vaginal laceration repair is intact, but you note a tense and tender 7-cm left vaginal wall hematoma. A CBC is normal except for a hematocrit of 22.2 (down from her predelivery hematocrit of 36). What is the most appropriate next step in this patient's management?

    A. Blood transfusion
    B. Incision and drainage of the hematoma with ligation of vessels and/or packing of the wound
    C. Sitz baths and iron replacement
    D. Administration of Pitocin
    E. Uterine artery embolization

161. A 16-year-old patient presents with intense genital itching for several days. She is sexually active with a new partner and otherwise healthy. She is afebrile, but exam reveals the specimen shown in Figure 161. You prescribe lindane shampoo and lotion, which successfully treats her infection. Which of the following genital infections is correctly matched to its causative agent?

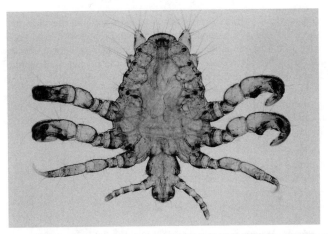

Figure 161 • Image courtesy of D. A. Burns, MB BS, FRCP, FRCP (Edin), Consultant Dermatologist and Honorary Senior Lecturer in Dermatology, Department of Dermatology, Leicester Royal Infirmary, Leicester, England.

    A. Crabs—*Phthirus pubis*
    B. Condyloma acuminata—human papillomavirus (HPV)
    C. Chancroid—L serotype of *Chlamydia trachomatis*
    D. Scabies—*Sarcoptes scabiei*
    E. Syphilis—*Haemophilus ducreyi*

162. A 27-year-old G_2P_2 who is postoperative day 5 from an uncomplicated, elective repeat low transverse cesarean section presents to the ED reporting copious light pink discharge from her wound. She denies fever or significant pain but is very anxious that the incision may be infected, as her husband noticed a small area where the wound seems to be separating. Physical exam is significant for an obese woman with a normal temperature and benign abdomen. However, the incision is quite moist and does appear to be separating on the right. You remove the steristrips and find that the wound separates with gentle probing, releasing moderate serosanguinous fluid. There is no erythema and moderate tenderness to your exam. Exploration of the wound reveals that the fascia is intact and the open wound tracks 3 cm to the left, is 4 cm deep, and is 4 cm long. What is the next best step in managing this woman's wound seroma?

A. Irrigate the wound and pack it with moist dressings
B. Administer antibiotics
C. Irrigate the wound and use steristrips to close it
D. Take her to the operating room for surgical closure of the wound
E. Expectant management

163. An obese 16-year-old girl presents to the ED complaining of diffuse abdominal pain of 6 hours duration. There is no associated nausea, vomiting, fever, chills, or anorexia. She denies any significant past medical or surgical history. You discover on exam that she is pregnant and contracting. On further questioning, she denies knowledge of the pregnancy and states that her LMP was "sometime last year." She denies substance use or trauma. Cervical exam reveals that she is 8 cm dilated with a bulging bag of water. You are able to visualize fetal cardiac motion on bedside US, confirm that the fetus is cephalic in presentation, and obtain fetal biometry that is consistent with approximately 38 weeks GA. Which of the following steps is appropriate for subsequent management of this patient?

A. Corticosteroids should be administered to promote fetal lung maturity
B. Magnesium tocolysis should be administered to stop labor
C. You should perform amniocentesis to assess fetal lung maturity
D. You should send the patient for formal US to get a better EGA
E. You should transfer the patient to labor and delivery for impending delivery

164. A 23-year-old G_1P_0 woman at 36 1/7 weeks GA presents to labor and delivery complaining of severe headache and visual changes. She has had an uneventful pregnancy until today. On exam, she appears mildly edematous and her BP is 159/91. She does not have any visual field defects and is slightly hyperreflexic. Fetal heart tones are reassuring, and there are no signs or symptoms of labor. Which of the following tests would assist in the diagnosis of mild preeclampsia?

A. CBC
B. Uric acid
C. Lactate dehydrogenase
D. Creatinine
E. 24-hour urine protein

165. An anxious 29-year-old nonpregnant woman comes to the ED reporting a 2-day history of copious, foul-smelling vaginal discharge that is green and frothy. She reports unprotected intercourse several days ago and is worried that she has contracted an STD. She is afebrile on exam and has a benign abdomen. Sterile speculum exam reveals an erythematous, punctate-appearing cervix and a large amount of discharge. You prepare the wet mount shown (Figure 165). There is no cervical motion tenderness, and the patient's uterus and adnexa are within normal limits. What is the diagnosis and appropriate management for this patient?

Figure 165 • Reproduced with permission from Axford J. Medicine. 2nd ed. Blackwell Publishing, 2004: Fig. 3.17, p. 87.

A. Bacterial vaginosis—metronidazole
B. Bacterial vaginosis—miconazole cream
C. Trichomonas—metronidazole
D. Trichomonas—miconazole cream
E. Candida vaginitis—miconazole cream

166. A 35-year-old G_3P_1 nonpregnant woman presents to the ED with fever and severe pelvic pain for 2 days. She is also experiencing mild nausea, but no emesis, dysuria, hematuria, anorexia, or changes in bowel movements. Significant past gynecological history includes sexual activity with a relatively new partner, sporadic condom usage, chlamydia as a teenager, hospitalization for PID several years ago, two elective first-trimester terminations, and one uncomplicated spontaneous vaginal delivery 7 years ago. She denies any medical or surgical history. Her temperature is 101.0°F, and she is in mild discomfort. Speculum exam is unremarkable, but bimanual exam reveals moderate cervical motion tenderness and a tender adnexal mass on her left side. Her WBC count returns as elevated with a left shift. You send the patient for US, which shows a somewhat loculated fluid collection/indistinct mass in the region of her right ovary and fallopian tube. What is the most likely diagnosis and appropriate next step in management?

A. Toxic shock syndrome (TSS)—inpatient IV antibiotics
B. Ovarian cancer—exploratory laparotomy and complete surgical staging
C. Tubo-ovarian abscess (TOA)/complex (TOC)—inpatient IV antibiotics
D. Tubo-ovarian abscess/complex—outpatient oral antibiotics
E. Endometritis—outpatient oral antibiotics

167. A 32-year-old G_0 woman presents to the ED with moderately severe left pelvic pain for 1 day. She denies fever, chills, trauma, weight changes, dysuria, or hematuria, but has experienced some mild nausea. She is about to start menstruating and reports that the same pain occurred at the beginning of her last few cycles. In addition to this worsening dysmenorrhea, her past gynecological history is significant for normal Pap smears and no STDs. She is sexually active with her husband, has mild dyspareunia, and does not use birth control as they have been trying unsuccessfully to conceive for approximately 1 year. A serum pregnancy test is negative, and she is afebrile with normal vital signs. Pertinent physical findings include a mildly tender lower abdomen, normal speculum exam, and bimanual exam revealing mild uterosacral nodularity and a small left adnexal mass that is tender to palpation. You send her for US, which reveals a 3-cm left adnexal mass that has a "ground glass" appearance (Figure 167). The remainder of the US is within normal limits. What is this patient's most likely diagnosis and how should she be treated?

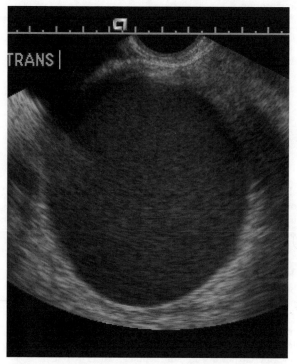

Figure 167 • Image provided by Departments of Radiology and Obstetrics & Gynecology, University of California, San Francisco.

 A. Endometriosis—expectant management and initiation of infertility evaluation
 B. Endometriosis—OCPs
 C. Ovarian cancer—exploratory laparotomy and complete cancer staging
 D. Mittelschmerz—NSAIDs
 E. Fibroids—hysterectomy

168. A 19-year-old G_1P_0 at 19 4/7 weeks GA presents to the ED with leakage of clear fluid noted upon awakening. She denies contractions, vaginal bleeding, fever, chills, or trauma. Pregnancy history is significant for entry into prenatal care at 17 weeks GA and diagnosis of chlamydia infection at that time, which was subsequently treated. Physical exam reveals a thin woman with normal temperature and nontender uterine fundus palpable 1 cm below the umbilicus. Sterile speculum exam shows pooling of vaginal fluid that is nitrazine positive and exhibits ferning under the microscope. Bedside US shows a live fetus in breech presentation. Which of the following measures would be appropriate management of preterm premature rupture of membranes (PPROM) in this patient?

A. Administration of corticosteroids for fetal lung maturity
B. Tocolysis
C. Administration of antibiotics
D. Induction of labor
E. Continuous fetal monitoring

169. A 33-year-old G_2P_1 woman at 29 2/7 weeks GA presents with severe right back pain radiating to her abdomen that began suddenly today. She denies prior episodes of pain, leakage of fluid, vaginal bleeding, fever, dysuria, hematuria, trauma, or drug usage. However, she does report some nausea and vomiting as well as mild contractions every 6 to 8 minutes. On exam, she is pacing the room, unable to stay still because of the pain. She is afebrile but with significant right CVAT. Fetal heart tones are reassuring, and tocometer reveals contractions every 5 to 8 minutes, but her cervix is closed, long, and high. A WBC count is within normal limits and urinalysis reveals microhematuria. What is the likely diagnosis and next step in management?

A. Nephrolithiasis—extracorporeal shock wave lithotripsy to break up large stones
B. Nephrolithiasis—IV hydration, pain control
C. Pyelonephritis—outpatient oral antibiotics
D. Pyelonephritis—inpatient IV antibiotics
E. Preterm labor—tocolysis

170. A 31-year-old G_1P_0 woman at 38 5/7 weeks GA with previously normal BPs reports to the ED after home monitoring reveals a BP of 158/98. She reports that the prenatal course has been uncomplicated. A repeat BP taken upon her arrival to the ED is 140/92, and the patient's urine dips 2+ proteinuria. Fetal heart rate (FHR) monitoring is reassuring. You draw the appropriate preeclamptic labs. As you await their return, the nurse informs you that the patient is having a seizure. Upon your arrival to the bedside, the patient is confused, but no longer seizing. Physical exam is within normal limits, and the lab results are still pending. An FHR tracing is obtained (Figure 170). Which of the following steps is the best management at this point?

A. Administer phenytoin
B. Administer diazepam
C. Administer phenobarbital
D. Administer magnesium sulfate
E. Emergent cesarean delivery

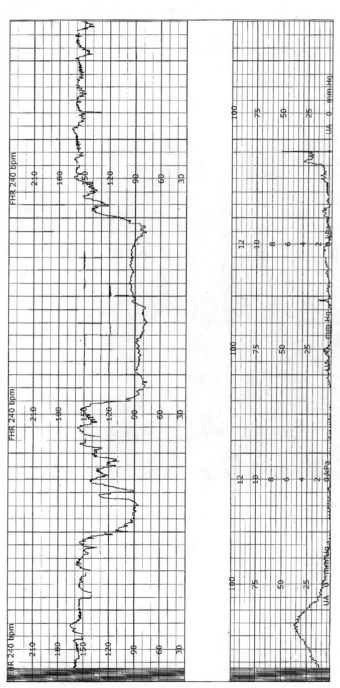

Figure 170 • Image provided by Department of Obstetrics & Gynecology, University of California, San Francisco.

171. A 42-year-old G₂P₂ woman comes to the ED reporting severe, burning pain in the genital area of 2 days duration. She has never experienced this pain before. Additionally, she reports a flu-like illness several days ago. Past medical and surgical histories are noncontributory. Her gynecological history is significant for two vaginal deliveries, regular menses, and normal Pap smears. She is sexually active with her boyfriend of 2 months and reports 100% condom usage. On exam, she is afebrile and does not have inguinal lymphadenopathy. You note several crops of vesicles and some ulcerated lesions on her perineum and labia majora that are exquisitely tender (Figure 171). What is the likely diagnosis and appropriate treatment?

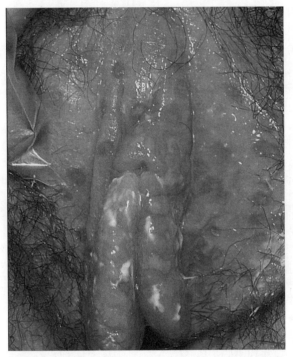

Figure 171 • Reproduced with permission from Callahan T. Blueprints Obstetrics & Gynecology. 3rd ed. Blackwell, 2004: Fig. 16-2, p. 149.

  A. Genital warts—imiquimod
  B. Genital warts—metronidazole
  C. *Molluscum contagiosum*—trichloroacetic acid
  D. Genital herpes—hydrocortisone cream
  E. Genital herpes—acyclovir

172. A 21-year-old G_1P_0 woman is brought to the ED by her friend, who reports that the patient has been experiencing persistent, severe vaginal bleeding since undergoing pregnancy termination 2 days prior via D&E of a 15-week gestation. She denies fever, chills, nausea, or vomiting, but does report painful cramping. The patient appears pale and is tachycardic with normal BP and temperature on exam. Her abdomen is benign, but speculum exam reveals a moderate amount of bleeding from her cervix, which appears to be open but intact. Bimanual exam is significant for a mildly tender 12-week-sized uterus, no cervical motion tenderness, and no adnexal masses or tenderness. You perform a bedside US and see that the uterus has a thick, heterogeneous endometrium (Figure 172), there is no free fluid in the pelvis, and both adnexa are within normal limits. What is the most likely diagnosis and appropriate treatment for this patient?

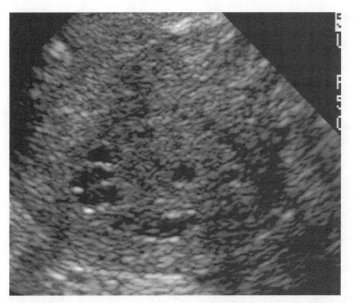

Figure 172 · Image provided by Departments of Radiology and Obstetrics & Gynecology, University of California, San Francisco.

    A. Retained POCs—suction curettage
    B. Retained POCs—expectant management
    C. Normal exam—expectant management
    D. Cervical laceration—operative repair
    E. Uterine perforation—diagnostic laparoscopy

173. A 28-year-old G_1P_0 woman at 19 0/7 weeks GA presents to the ED complaining of pelvic pressure and increased vaginal discharge. She denies cramps or contractions, leakage of fluid, vaginal bleeding, or fever. Her pregnancy has been uncomplicated thus far. She had two prenatal visits at 8 and 14 weeks and is scheduled to see her provider again after her routine US appointment scheduled for tomorrow. Her past gynecological history is significant for a cone biopsy of the cervix at age 23 for persistent high-grade squamous intraepithelial lesion (HSIL). All subsequent Pap smears have been within normal limits. Speculum exam reveals a cervix that is approximately 2 cm dilated with visible amniotic membranes. You also notice a pool of fluid in the vagina, which is nitrazine and fern positive. Which of the following statements is true regarding the management of this patient's incompetent cervix?

A. Her risk factors for incompetent cervix include her Pap smear in the first trimester
B. Treatment options include emergent cerclage placement
C. Patients with a history of incompetent cervix can be offered a prophylactic cerclage in subsequent pregnancies that should be placed prior to conception
D. Treatment options include pregnancy termination
E. Her incompetent cervix could have been diagnosed by US at 14 weeks

174. A 70-year-old demented woman is sent from her nursing home to the ED when she is found to have vaginal bleeding. Review of her medical records reveals that she has hypertension and suffered a cerebrovascular accident 2 years prior with subsequent speech and motor deficits, necessitating full-time care. She never had any children and became menopausal at age 52. On exam, she is awake, but demented and unable to communicate. Gynecological exam reveals a large, necrotic, bleeding sore on her left vulva. Additionally, she has left inguinal lymphadenopathy. Her uterus is not palpable on bimanual exam, but you confirm its presence as well as the absence of adnexal masses on US. The vaginal tissue is atrophied but otherwise within normal limits for her age. You suspect a vulvar malignancy. Which of the following statements is true regarding cancer of the vulva?

A. Vulvar cancer is one of the most common gynecologic malignancies
B. Symptoms of vulvar cancer include bleeding, pain, pruritus, ascites, and bloating
C. Malignant melanoma is the most common subtype of vulvar cancer
D. Treatment of squamous cell cancer of the vulva involves wide local excision with lymph node dissection
E. Staging of vulvar cancer can be performed via biopsy of the mass and palpation of the inguinal lymph nodes

175. A 33-year-old G_3P_2 woman who had an uncomplicated delivery of an infant 3 weeks ago presents to the ED complaining of right breast pain and fever for 2 days. On physical exam, you note an area of focal tenderness, warmth, and erythema on the right breast. The patient is found to have a temperature of 101.2°F and an elevated WBC count of 12,000. Which of the following is appropriate treatment for mastitis?

A. Symptomatic treatment of pain with acetaminophen only
B. Stop breastfeeding until completion of antibiotic course
C. Oral dicloxacillin
D. IV antibiotics
E. Oral doxycycline

176. A 23-year-old G$_0$ woman presents with acute-onset, severe right lower quadrant pain and mild nausea. She denies fever, chills, or vaginal bleeding or discharge. The patient reports feeling this pain twice in the last 6 months, with this time being the worst it has ever been. On physical exam, she is afebrile, appears extremely uncomfortable, and has severe RLQ tenderness, but does not have any peritoneal signs. Pelvic exam is significant for a tender right adnexal mass and cervical motion tenderness. Pelvic US reveals minimal fluid in the cul-de-sac and a 6 cm right adnexal mass with no Doppler flow (Figure 176). The patient's WBC count and hematocrit are normal, and a urine pregnancy test is negative. Which of the following is the most likely diagnosis?

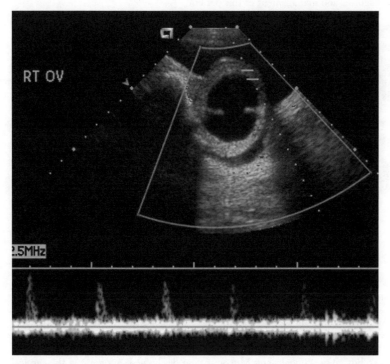

Figure 176 • Image provided by Departments of Radiology and Obstetrics & Gynecology, University of California, San Francisco.

    A. Acute appendicitis
    B. Early ectopic pregnancy
    C. Torsion of adnexa
    D. PID
    E. Ruptured hemorrhagic ovarian cyst

177. A 27-year-old woman presents to the ED with complaints of heavy vaginal bleeding and painful abdominal cramping that started this morning. She reports that she stopped taking birth control pills approximately 3 months ago in an effort to conceive and that she had some light spotting a month later but no normal menstrual period since then. Her blood type is O positive, and her hematocrit is 39.2. A urine pregnancy test in the ED is positive. On physical exam, you note mild lower abdominal tenderness in the midline, but an otherwise benign abdominal exam. On speculum exam, you note a large amount of bright red blood in the vaginal vault and an open cervical os containing large blood clots. Endovaginal US (Figure 177) confirms the presence of a gestational sac in the uterus consistent with a 6-week gestation, but no yolk sac is visible. What is the correct diagnosis and management of this patient?

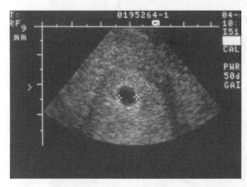

Figure 177 • Image provided by Departments of Radiology and Obstetrics & Gynecology, University of California, San Francisco.

A. Ectopic pregnancy—emergent surgery
B. Threatened abortion—D&C
C. Incomplete abortion—expectant management
D. Inevitable abortion—D&C
E. Complete abortion—expectant management

178. A 20-year-old G_1P_1 woman presents to the ED complaining of nausea, vomiting, and lower abdominal pain for the past 2 days. She reports intermittent condom usage with her partner of 3 months. Her vital signs are within normal limits, with the exception of a temperature of 100.2°F. On exam, you note abdominal, adnexal, and cervical motion tenderness, but no peritoneal signs. Mucopurulent discharge is apparent at the cervical os. A urine pregnancy test is negative, and the patient's WBC count is 13,700/mm³. A wet mount shows numerous leukocytes. Which of the following is an absolute indication for inpatient treatment of PID?

A. Age greater than 18
B. Age less than 40
C. Severe nausea and vomiting
D. Adnexal tenderness
E. Penicillin allergy

179. A 28-year-old G_3P_0 woman is brought to the ED shortly after passing out. She is conscious on arrival, but appears to be in acute distress and severe pain. She reports vaginal bleeding and worsening left lower abdominal pain that became sharp and severe just prior to her loss of consciousness. She had a positive urine pregnancy test 4 weeks ago and is certain that her LMP was 8 weeks ago. Past medical history is significant for PID that was treated 5 years ago. Her vital signs are BP 84/40, pulse 118, respiration 26, and temperature 97.2°F. Urine pregnancy test is positive. The patient has a normal WBC count and a hematocrit of 32.3. On physical exam, she has diffuse lower abdominal pain and exhibits guarding and rebound. Pelvic exam reveals cervical motion tenderness and significant tenderness to palpation in the left adnexal region. Transvaginal US (Figure 179) shows a large amount of free fluid in the cul-de-sac, but no masses and no intrauterine pregnancy. What is the most appropriate next step in managing this patient?

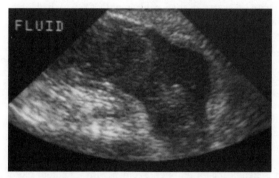

Figure 179 • Image provided by Departments of Radiology and Obstetrics & Gynecology, University of California, San Francisco.

A. Uterine curettage to definitively exclude ectopic pregnancy
B. Perform a culdocentesis
C. Obtain a quantitative β-hCG level to determine whether medical or surgical treatment is indicated
D. Administer methotrexate and follow serial quantitative β-hCG levels for appropriate decline
E. Stabilize the patient and take her emergently to the operating room

180. A 20-year-old G_0 woman presents to the ED in tears. She reports being sexually assaulted by three men unknown to her while attending a party this evening. You obtain a history from her, which is difficult because she is visibly shaken and upset. She doesn't believe any of the assailants used a condom and is unsure whether they ejaculated. There was no oral or anal penetration. On speculum exam, you obtain swabs from the vagina for evidence and for microscopic exam. You do not see any evidence of spermatozoa, trichomonads, or bacterial vaginosis. Which of the following steps would be appropriate management of this patient?

A. Start oral contraceptive pills immediately
B. Azithromycin 1 g PO and ceftriaxone 250 mg IM × 1
C. Do not contact police if the patient does not want to press charges
D. Reassure her that she has no risk of pregnancy
E. Reassure her that she has minimal risk of contracting HIV if there was no ejaculation

181. A 17-year-old G_0 woman is brought to the ED by her mother, who is concerned that the patient has been experiencing fevers, rigors, nausea, vomiting, and myalgias since this morning. She is not sexually active, and her LMP began 5 days ago. Her vital signs are BP 84/46, temperature 103.1°F, pulse 122, and respiration 24. On physical exam, the patient appears acutely ill, has a diffuse erythematous rash, and exhibits mild, diffuse abdominal tenderness, but no nuchal rigidity. After removal of a blood-saturated tampon, pelvic exam reveals a small amount of blood in the vaginal vault but no cervical motion tenderness or vaginal discharge, and the uterus and adnexa are within normal limits. Laboratory studies are significant for a WBC count of 21,000, platelets of 93,000, and elevated BUN and creatinine. Which of the following statements about this patient's diagnosis is true?

A. It is caused by *Streptococcus agalactiae*
B. It has been associated with polycystic ovarian syndrome (PCOS), vaginal infections, vaginal and cesarean delivery, and postpartum endometritis
C. Blood cultures are often positive
D. Treatment may include admission to an intensive care unit for management of hypotension
E. There are approximately 1500 cases per year in the United States

182. A 27-year-old G_2P_1 woman at 35 1/7 weeks GA presents to OB triage and anxiously states that she has not felt the baby move for the past 5 hours. She denies vaginal bleeding, rupture of membranes, or uterine contractions. The pregnancy is complicated by poorly controlled gestational diabetes mellitus requiring insulin administration. The patient began twice-weekly antepartum testing at 32 weeks GA, but has missed several appointments. Physical exam is significant for an obese woman with a random blood glucose of 154. Her cervical exam is 1 cm dilated, 50% effaced, and −3 station. Non-stress testing is performed (Figure 182). What is the most appropriate next step in the management of this high-risk patient with decreased fetal movement?

A. Administer insulin to decrease the patient's glucose level
B. Vibroacoustic stimulation (VAS) of the fetus followed by US to look for gross and fine fetal movements
C. Administer betamethasone to promote fetal lung maturity in anticipation of possible premature delivery
D. Begin induction of labor with a prostaglandin agent
E. Emergent cesarean section

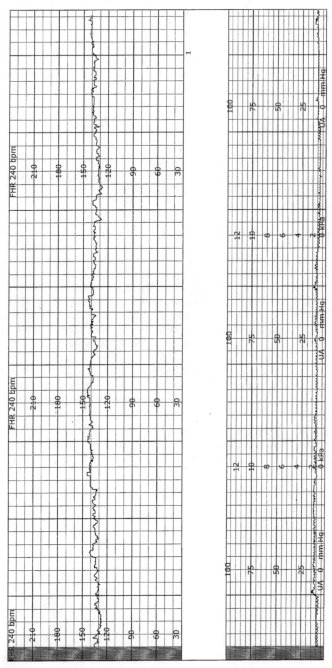

Figure 182 · Image provided by Department of Obstetrics & Gynecology, University of California, San Francisco.

183. A 32-year-old G_3P_3 woman presents to the ED complaining of persistent fevers and abdominal pain that have worsened over the past day and are only temporarily relieved by ibuprofen. She is postpartum day 7 after a vaginal delivery of a term infant male weighing 3500 g. The delivery was complicated by a postpartum hemorrhage requiring manual extraction of the placenta. The patient's vaginal bleeding has decreased since discharge from the hospital, requiring two to four pad changes per day. Her vital signs are BP 108/72, temperature 102.6°F, pulse 96, and respiration 20. On physical exam, she has fundal tenderness but no peritoneal signs. Pelvic exam confirms uterine tenderness and reveals scant vaginal bleeding as well as a minimal amount of purulent discharge. The laceration repair is intact and hemostatic. Laboratory studies reveal a hematocrit of 34.4 and a WBC count of 18,000 with a left shift. What is the appropriate diagnosis and treatment for this patient?

A. Delayed postpartum hemorrhage—D&C
B. Placenta accreta—exploratory laparotomy
C. Undiagnosed vaginal hematoma—ligation of the offending blood vessel
D. Endomyometritis—clindamycin and gentamicin
E. Endomyometritis—D&C

184. A 30-year-old G_0 woman presents to the ED after an episode of postcoital bleeding that soaked a pad over the last 2 hours. She reports four to five prior episodes of postcoital bleeding over the last few months that were less severe. She denies any significant past medical history. Her menses occur every month and are regular. She has not had a Pap smear since age 18, when she first became sexually active. At that time, she was found to have chlamydia, for which she underwent treatment. The patient reports multiple current sexual partners, and she uses condoms intermittently. Her hematocrit is 40.1. Vital signs and physical exam are within normal limits. Pelvic exam reveals a minimal amount of blood and watery discharge in the vaginal vault, as well as a 2 cm × 3 cm exophytic mass on the cervix that does not appear to involve the upper vagina or fornix. The uterus and adnexa are within normal limits. You biopsy the lesion, which returns 1 week later as cervical cancer invasive to 7 mm. The patient undergoes staging, which reveals negative cystoscopy, proctoscopy, and IV pyelogram (IVP). What is the stage and appropriate treatment of her disease?

A. Ib1—cone biopsy to preserve fertility
B. Ib1—radical hysterectomy or radiation therapy
C. Ib2—radical hysterectomy or radiation therapy
D. IIa—radical hysterectomy
E. IIb—radiation therapy

185. A 34-year-old G$_4$P$_3$ woman at 33 4/7 weeks GA presents to the ED complaining of a gush of vaginal bleeding as well as the onset of severely painful uterine contractions. The patient denies history of abdominal trauma, recent intercourse, or cocaine usage and has a history of three prior vaginal deliveries. Her vital signs are BP 162/99, temperature 98.4°F, pulse 114, and respiration 18. Physical exam reveals a woman in moderate distress with a firm and tender uterus. The fetal heart rate (FHR) tracing is initially formally reactive, with a baseline rate of approximately 145 beats per minutes (bpm). US exam confirms that there is no evidence of placenta previa. On sterile speculum exam, a moderate amount of blood is seen in the vaginal vault. Cervical exam reveals 1 1/2-cm dilation, 50% effacement, and –3 station. As you are writing the patient's note, the nurse informs you that the FHR tracing now shows a prolonged deceleration of 5 minutes duration to approximately 80 bpm with no signs of spontaneous recovery to baseline (Figure 185). The nurse has already turned the patient to her left side, given O$_2$ by face mask, and checked her BP, which is now 158/102. What is the most appropriate next step in this patient's management?

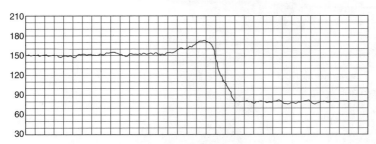

Figure 185 · Reproduced with permission from Caughey A. Blueprints Q&A Step 3 Obstetrics & Gynecology. 1st ed. Blackwell Science, 2002: Fig. 89, p. 55.

A. Transfuse 2 units of packed red blood cells (PRBC) immediately and have the lab type and cross 2 additional units

B. Administer betamethasone to promote fetal lung maturity in anticipation of preterm delivery

C. Administer magnesium sulfate tocolysis to alleviate the fetal distress from contractions

D. Initiate induction of labor for nonreassuring FHR tracing

E. Move to the operating room (OR) for cesarean section for nonreassuring FHR tracing

186. A 36-year-old G_2P_2 woman presents to the ED with acute-onset shortness of breath and chest pain. She is 1 day postpartum following a cesarean delivery and left the hospital prior to the recommended day of discharge (generally, postoperative day 2 or 3) due to childcare issues. Of note, the patient is not breastfeeding. She denies a history of trauma. Her past medical history is significant for obesity, and her vital signs are BP 116/74, temperature 100.0°F, pulse 112, respiration 28, and O_2 saturation 91% on room air. On physical exam, she is in moderate distress, is tachypneic, and has rales and mildly decreased breath sounds in the left lung. Pelvic exam reveals a minimal amount of blood in the vaginal vault but is otherwise within normal limits. Chest X-ray is negative, but EKG reveals sinus tachycardia and nonspecific ST-T wave changes. A blood gas drawn on room air reveals an a-A gradient of 43. You order a ventilation/perfusion (V/Q) scan, which is read as inconclusive. At this point, a pulmonary arteriogram is performed (Figure 186). Which of the following would be the most appropriate treatment for this patient?

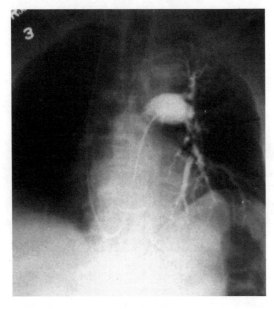

Figure 186 • Reproduced with permission from Dildy G. Critical Care Obstetrics. Blackwell Science, 2004: Fig. 20-7, p. 284.

A. Supplemental oxygen by nasal cannula
B. IV heparin
C. Low-molecular-weight heparin
D. Oral warfarin therapy
E. IV furosemide

187. A 68-year-old G_0 woman with a history of stage IIIc ovarian cancer presents to the ED with persistent nausea and vomiting for several days. She has not had anything to eat or drink for 2 days. Additionally, she has not had a bowel movement or passed gas in 5 days. Approximately 7 months ago, she underwent TAH-BSO, complete staging work-up, and 6 cycles of chemotherapy for her ovarian cancer. Her vital signs are BP 114/72, temperature 100.8°F, pulse 108, and respiration 18. On physical exam, she is a thin, obtunded woman with dry mucous membranes and skin tenting. Abdominal exam reveals distention, absent bowel sounds, severe tenderness, and peritoneal signs.

Laboratory studies are significant for a hematocrit of 45.2 and WBC of 15,000. You send the patient for an abdominal X-ray series, which reveals numerous air-fluid levels and a sliver of hyperlucency below the diaphragm. What is the next step in the management of this patient?

A. Insert a nasogastric tube (NGT) and expectant management
B. Begin total parenteral nutrition (TPN)
C. Laparoscopy to look for residual disease
D. Administer broad-spectrum antibiotics and plan laparotomy when her signs of infection have resolved
E. Proceed to the operating room (OR) for exploratory laparotomy

188. A 36-year-old G_0 woman presents to the ED complaining of severe pelvic pain for 2 days. The patient is well known to you and has endometriosis confirmed by laparoscopy. She denies history of current or past physical or sexual abuse and does not desire future fertility. Over the past 3 years, she has tried various treatment regimens, including both cyclic and continuous OCPs. The latter yielded a 4-month pain-free period. The patient admits to recent discontinuation of the continuous OCPs secondary to concern regarding amenorrhea. Her vital signs are stable, and she is afebrile. Physical exam reveals normal bowel sounds, mild pelvic tenderness, but no masses or peritoneal signs. On pelvic exam, the patient has diffuse pelvic tenderness and uterosacral nodularity on rectovaginal exam. There are no adnexal masses or vaginal discharge or bleeding. Pelvic US is within normal limits. Which of the following steps is the most appropriate treatment for this patient?

A. Resume cyclic OCPs
B. Resume continuous OCPs
C. Trial of progestin treatment
D. Trial of GnRH agonist treatment
E. Exploratory laparoscopy

189. An 18-year-old G_1P_0 woman at 14 4/7 weeks GA presents to the ED complaining of weight loss and severe nausea and vomiting for 3 days. This is her fifth visit to the ED for this problem, and she has had two prior short-term hospitalizations. She has tried vitamin B_6, Reglan (metoclopramide), Tigan (trimethobenzamide), and Compazine (prochlorperazine), but obtained only temporary relief. She has no significant past medical history but is currently in an abusive relationship with the father of the baby. Her vital signs are BP 102/68, temperature 96.8°F, pulse 96, and respiration 16. On physical exam, she appears uncomfortable, has dry mucous membranes, and shows poor skin turgor. Pelvic exam is within normal limits. Laboratory studies reveal hypokalemia, hypochloremia, alkalemia, hematocrit of 48, and a BUN/creatinine ratio exceeding 20:1. Urinalysis reveals ketones and high specific gravity. Which of the following components of this patient's management should be used only when the others have failed?

A. Hospitalization for IV hydration and repletion of electrolytes
B. Social work consultation
C. Zofran (ondansetron) 4 mg IV, then 8 mg PO TID when tolerating oral intake
D. Initiation of total parenteral nutrition (TPN)
E. Placement of a nasogastric feeding tube

190. A 31-year-old G_2P_2 woman presents to the ED complaining of severe abdominal pain and vaginal spotting. She denies fever, chills, nausea, and vomiting. Over the past 6 months, she has noticed that the duration and amount of her regular menses have diminished. This is coincident with the fact that approximately 6 months ago, she underwent a loop electrosurgical excision procedure (LEEP) for cervical dysplasia. Her vital signs and physical exam are within normal limits. On pelvic exam, you note a slightly enlarged, tender, anteverted, and anteflexed uterus with cervical motion tenderness and no cervical, uterine, or adnexal masses. What are the most likely diagnosis and appropriate treatment?

A. Pelvic abscess—CT-guided drainage
B. Endometriosis—diagnostic laparoscopy
C. Progression of residual cervical dysplasia to cancer—hysterectomy
D. Cervical stenosis—OCPs
E. Cervical stenosis—cervical dilatation

191. A 24-year-old G_1P_0 woman who had a positive urine pregnancy test 9 weeks ago presents to the ED complaining of severe nausea, vomiting, and painless vaginal bleeding. She has not had her initial prenatal exam yet. She denies any significant past medical history. On physical exam, she has no abdominal tenderness, but her fundus is palpable just below the umbilicus. Pelvic exam reveals a small amount of tissue at the cervical os, but no lesion, discharge, or active bleeding. Quantitative β-hCG is 117,000. US is performed (Figure 191). Which of the following statements is correct regarding this patient's diagnosis and management?

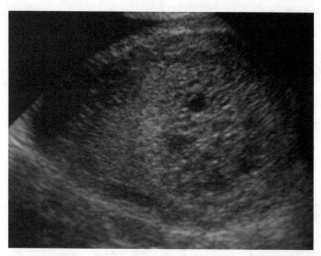

Figure 191 · Image provided by Departments of Radiology and Obstetrics & Gynecology, University of California, San Francisco.

A. Tissue evacuated from the uterine cavity is likely to have a 46,XX karyotype.
B. Treatment should be expectant management.
C. Treatment should be hysterectomy.
D. Treatment should be immediate single-agent chemotherapy.
E. There is a 25% risk of recurrence with subsequent pregnancies.

192. A 62-year-old G_3P_3 woman presents to the ED 5 days after undergoing a laparoscopic Burch culposuspension procedure for stress urinary incontinence. She reports that she has been able to micturate only small volumes over the past 6 hours despite constant urgency. Additionally, she is experiencing mild nausea and increasing midline lower abdominal pain without radiation, but denies vomiting, fever, chills, constipation, or loose stools. Her past medical history is noncontributory. Vital signs are within normal limits. On physical exam, you note mild suprapubic pain, normal bowel sounds, and no peritoneal signs. Pelvic exam reveals discomfort with uterine manipulation, but no cervical motion tenderness, no vaginal discharge or bleeding, and no uterine, cervical, or adnexal masses. Rectal exam is nontender with normal tone. You collect a 20-cc urine specimen, which gives the following results on urine dipstick: specific gravity 1.010, no RBCs, negative leukocyte esterase, 2 to 5 bacteria/high-power field, and 1 to 3 squamous cells/high-power field. Which of the following is the most appropriate next step in management of this patient?

A. Outpatient treatment of UTI
B. Hospitalization for IV antibiotic treatment
C. Straight catheterization to obtain a clean sample for urinalysis
D. Placement of a Foley catheter
E. Surgical exploration/repair

193. You are called by an ED resident to evaluate a 26-year-old G_4P_2 woman presenting with epigastric pain and severe nausea. On arrival to the ER, her BP is 155/110, her heart rate is 72, and her temperature is 37.6°C. The patient reports that she has missed her last three menstrual periods (and normally has very regular cycles). A urine pregnancy test is positive, and urine dipstick demonstrates 2+ protein but is otherwise normal. A CBC with platelets, LFTs, amylase, and lipase was sent immediately and all values were within normal limits. Abdominal US in the ER showed no evidence of appendicitis or cholestatic disease. The resident is not sure what she is seeing when scanning the uterus. Before hanging up, she asks if any laboratory values should be added on to her original orders to help evaluate this patient. Serum levels of which *one* of the following would be *most* valuable in the diagnosis of this patient?

A. CA-125
B. Quantitative β-hCG
C. Magnesium
D. Alpha-fetoprotein (AFP)
E. Thyroxine (T_4)

194. A 38-year-old G_1P_0 woman presents to the ED at 9 weeks GA with 2 days of vaginal bleeding. She is very upset about the possibility of miscarriage, as this is a highly desired pregnancy achieved with intrauterine insemination. An US at 7 weeks was thought to show a normal intrauterine pregnancy. Pelvic exam in the emergency room reveals vesicles protruding from the cervical os and a small amount of active bleeding. Pelvic US reveals a thickened placenta with multiple cysts and a fetus consistent with her dating. Quantitative β-hCG is 183,000. If suction evacuation is performed, what will be the most likely karyotype of the tissue recovered?

A. 46,XX
B. 47,XXY
C. 47,XX+18
D. 47,XX+21
E. 69,XXY

195. A 30-year-old G_0 female comes into the ED complaining of extreme pelvic pain. The pain began insidiously over the last few days. The patient reports a prior history of similar pain, but this time the pain is worse. It seems to coincide with her periods, and she has noticed increasing pain with intercourse. The patient has been married for 4 years and, despite not using contraception, has been unable to conceive. A urine serum pregnancy test is negative. The patient's pelvic exam is unremarkable except for diffuse pain of both adnexa. A pelvic US reveals a normal midline uterus with a slightly thickened endometrium consistent with current menstruation. Also, two 6-cm well-circumscribed masses with low attenuation are identified, one in each adnexa. The patient tells you that she has spoken with her doctor in the past about a diagnostic laparoscopy to evaluate the etiology of this pain. Which of the following potential intraoperative findings is the most likely cause of her pain?

A. Corpus luteum cyst
B. Scant powder-burn lesions
C. Bilateral endometriomas (chocolate cysts)
D. Peritoneal tuberculosis implants
E. Tubo-ovarian abscess (TOA)

196. You are called from the ED about a pregnant patient in the first trimester presenting with a febrile illness and history of a recent new sexual contact. The physician's assistant asks about the risk of transmission of various infections during pregnancy while the lab work is pending. You inform him that which of the following infections has been shown to be unlikely to be transmitted across the placenta?

A. Toxoplasmosis
B. HIV
C. *Neisseria gonorrhoeae*
D. Varicella zoster virus
E. Parvovirus

197. A 19-year-old G_0 woman presents to the ED several hours after experiencing a sudden sharp pain in the left lower quadrant that has subsided over the last few hours and become more diffuse. Her LMP was approximately 2 weeks ago. She reports similar prior episodes of pain on the right side 2 to 3 months ago, has been sexually active with the same partner for 2 years, and denies vaginal discharge. She is afebrile, has a normal white count, and has a negative urine pregnancy test. On physical exam, she has mild diffuse abdominal pain, but no peritoneal signs. Pelvic exam is within normal limits with no cervical motion tenderness. What is the most likely diagnosis?

A. Mittelschmerz
B. PID
C. Adnexal torsion
D. Ruptured ectopic pregnancy
E. Appendicitis

198. A 17-year-old G_3P_1 woman at 32 5/7 weeks GA presents to the ED complaining of moderately painful uterine contractions every 5 minutes for the past hour. Significant prenatal issues include obesity (prepregnancy weight of 253 lb), history of a prior preterm delivery at 32 weeks gestation, and history of a therapeutic abortion at 11 weeks gestation 3 years ago. Her vital signs are stable, and the patient is afebrile. On physical exam, she is an obese woman in moderate discomfort but with an otherwise negative exam. Sterile speculum exam and wet mount reveal abundant pseudohyphae, and cervical exam reveals 3-cm dilation and 75% effacement. Which of the following is this patient's biggest risk factor for preterm delivery?

A. Prior preterm delivery
B. Prior therapeutic abortion (TAB)
C. Vaginal candidiasis
D. Prepregnancy weight
E. Maternal age

199. A 31-year-old woman presents to the ED complaining of gradual-onset left lower quadrant pain. She denies nausea, vomiting, fever, chills, constipation, or loose stools. However, she notes an 8-lb weight gain over the past month. Her gynecological history is significant for current infertility treatment by ovulation induction with gonadotropins. During her infertility work-up, a hysterosalpingogram revealed an occluded left tube, and laparoscopy revealed stage 3 endometriosis. The patient reports that she has continued to have unprotected intercourse throughout her current treatment. However, her urine pregnancy test is negative. Her vital signs are within normal limits. On physical exam, you note mild abdominal distention, tenderness to palpation in the left lower quadrant, and a left adnexal mass. No blood or discharge is apparent in the vaginal vault, and exam fails to show any cervical motion tenderness. US exam reveals an enlarged ovary approximately 7 cm × 8 cm in size that is composed of numerous enlarged follicles. There is a moderate amount of free fluid in the cul-de-sac. The patient's hematocrit is 42 and her WBC count is 8000. What is this patient's most likely diagnosis?

A. Adnexal torsion
B. Ovarian hyperstimulation (OHSS)
C. Early ectopic pregnancy
D. Endometrioma
E. PID

200. A 29-year-old G_2P_0 woman at 10 2/7 weeks GA by a sure LMP presents to the ED reporting cramping that started this afternoon. She is very anxious because she had a miscarriage with her last pregnancy and this pregnancy is highly desired. The patient denies vaginal bleeding, usage of an IUD, history of pelvic infections, smoking, or ectopic pregnancy. On exam, she is tearful but otherwise appears well with normal vital signs. Her abdomen is soft, nontender, and without masses. On speculum exam, no blood is seen in the vaginal vault. Bimanual exam reveals a mildly enlarged, nontender uterus, no cervical motion tenderness or dilation, and no adnexal masses or tenderness. A bedside US (Figure 200) reveals an intrauterine gestational sac with a fetal pole consistent in size with a 6-week gestation but no cardiac motion and no adnexal masses or free fluid in the cul-de-sac. A quantitative β-hCG is 13,327. Which of the following statements is true regarding this patient's diagnosis and treatment?

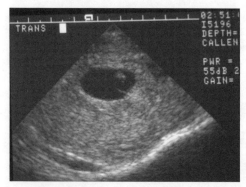

Figure 200 • Image provided by Departments of Radiology and Obstetrics & Gynecology, University of California, San Francisco.

A. She has experienced a complete abortion
B. Expectant management is not appropriate
C. She can be given a prostaglandin to induce uterine evacuation
D. RhoGAM should be administered
E. She should be evaluated for recurrent pregnancy loss

Answer Key

151. E	168. D	185. E
152. B	169. B	186. B
153. D	170. D	187. E
154. E	171. E	188. B
155. C	172. A	189. D
156. B	173. D	190. E
157. B	174. D	191. A
158. E	175. C	192. D
159. A	176. C	193. B
160. B	177. D	194. E
161. B	178. C	195. C
162. A	179. E	196. C
163. E	180. B	197. A
164. E	181. D	198. A
165. C	182. B	199. B
166. C	183. D	200. C
167. A	184. B	

151. **E.** Appendicitis is the diagnosis most consistent with this patient's clinical history, acute abdomen, fever, and leukocytosis. Of note, the enlarged uterus can displace the appendix, making McBurney's point an unreliable landmark in pregnant women. Exploratory laparotomy is the most appropriate treatment for suspected appendicitis in pregnancy, as laparoscopy would be unsafe and technically difficult with the gravid uterus.

A. Diverticulosis is generally a condition of older age and occurs uncommonly in women of child-bearing age. Additionally, diverticuli do not cause an acute abdomen and are typically symptomatic only when inflamed (i.e., diverticulitis). Treatment would involve dietary changes and stool softeners.

B. This patient is having focal abdominal pain, which is inconsistent with contractions. While it is important to rule out the diagnosis of preterm labor, this patient has no identifiable contractions on tocometer and a closed cervix that is not effaced. At 33 weeks GA, treatment of preterm labor would involve tocolysis and administration of corticosteroids to promote fetal lung maturity.

C. In general, patients with pain due to nephrolithiasis (i.e., renal colic) are constantly moving, whereas patients with an acute abdomen lie as still as possible. Such patients will often have microscopic or gross hematuria on urinalysis. The more important diagnosis to rule out in this patient with fever, vomiting, abdominal pain, and leukocytosis is pyelonephritis. The lack of bacteria and WBCs on urinalysis and no CVAT make this a less likely diagnosis.

D. Placental abruption, which involves the premature separation of the normally implanted placenta, can result in severe hemorrhage and fetal death. It typically occurs in the third trimester and involves vaginal bleeding associated with severe abdominal pain and/or frequent contractions; bleeding can also be concealed, however. This patient is not having any vaginal bleeding, contractions, or evidence of nonreassuring fetal status. Immediate delivery would be indicated in the event of massive placental abruption.

152. **B.** This patient's symptoms are concerning for HELLP syndrome (hemolysis, elevated liver enzymes, low platelets), which is a subcategory of severe preeclampsia. Affected patients can also develop disseminated intravascular coagulation. Unlike in mild and severe preeclampsia, hypertension and proteinuria are not always present in HELLP syndrome. Diagnosis is therefore made via clinical suspicion and a finding of the lab abnormalities that make up the syndrome's name. HELLP syndrome is uncommon, but can involve rapid maternal and fetal deterioration. Treatment involves magnesium sulfate seizure prophylaxis and delivery. In this patient at term and already in early labor, vaginal delivery would be the optimal choice.

A, D. Epigastric pain, nausea, and vomiting can be suggestive of pancreatitis or some other GI etiology, in which case IV fluids and pain control would likely be appropriate initial therapy. However, this patient's pain is not related to food intake. GI etiology can be considered, but the more important diagnosis of HELLP syndrome must first be ruled out.

C. Tocolysis is not indicated in this patient at term whose signs and symptoms are concerning for severe illness.

E. See the explanation for B. The optimal mode of delivery would be vaginal rather than surgical in a patient with a potential for hemodynamic instability and coagulopathy. In the event of rapid deterioration remote from delivery, however, operative delivery may be necessary.

153. **D.** US shows mild to moderate amounts of free fluid in the pelvis, but no evidence of adnexal (not shown) or uterine masses. This patient's sudden pain occurring in the midluteal phase that is now resolving in the setting of an essentially normal physical exam and lab studies is most consistent with a ruptured ovarian cyst. Her abdominal discomfort is most likely due to peritoneal irritation by the free fluid. In a hemodynamically stable patient, treatment involves pain relief and outpatient follow-up. It is also reasonable to observe the patient with serial blood counts to confirm that she is not having continued bleeding. Follicular cysts are common functional cysts found in women of reproductive age. They result from the failure of a developing follicle to rupture and generally resolve within 60 days. However, they can grow to a size of 8 cm and are subject to torsion as well as rupture, both of which can cause pain.

A. Diagnostic laparoscopy is not indicated in a patient without an acute abdomen.

B. This patient does not show evidence of infection or findings consistent with PID or tubo-ovarian abscess. Antibiotics are therefore not indicated.

C. A GI etiology is unlikely in this patient without any GI symptoms and an US exam consistent with a ruptured ovarian cyst.

E. This patient is not experiencing vaginal bleeding or other signs or symptoms that would necessitate a D&C of the uterus.

154. **E.** This patient's symptoms are suggestive of a UTI, which is one of the most common infections of the lower GU tract. UTIs occur more commonly in women than in men due to the relatively shorter length of the urethra in women. All of the items listed in this answer choice are possible findings in the setting of UTI. Nitrites are produced by bacteria. The presence of WBCs is suggestive of infection, and leukocyte esterase is suggestive of the presence of WBCs. RBCs can be present in urine due to inflammation and irritation of bladder or urethral mucosa.

A. While WBCs can be seen in UTIs, lipids are not a typical component of a urinalysis (or UTIs).

B. WBCs and calcium deposits might be seen with nephrolithiasis or renal stones.

C, D. Renal epithelium can be seen in urine specimens in the setting of renal disease, but are generally not present with an uncomplicated lower UTI.

155. **C.** This patient appears to have an uncomplicated UTI. She is afebrile and does not have any CVAT, which might be suggestive of pyelonephritis. Treatment for UTIs should include oral antibiotics and fluid intake. UTIs are often caused by GI organisms such as *E. coli*, *S. saprophyticus*, and *Enterococcus*. Common oral regimens for UTIs include Macrodantin (nitrofurantoin), Bactrim (trimethoprim-sulfamethoxazole), Keflex (cephalexin), and ampicillin. Additionally, urine should be cultured to identify the infectious organism and assess its sensitivity to antibiotics to ensure appropriate treatment.

A. Fluid intake is an important part of maintaining adequate hydration and ensuring that antibiotics reach the lower urinary tract.

B. There is no indication for a Foley catheter. Occasionally in patients who have primary genital HSV infection, the dysuria is so great that they will need a catheter placed. This patient's symptoms can be treated with phenazopyridine (Pyridium), which acts as a topical analgesic by becoming concentrated in the urine.

D. If a patient has signs and symptoms concerning for pyelonephritis and cannot tolerate oral intake, she should be admitted for IV antibiotics. Otherwise, oral antibiotics will rapidly and adequately treat uncomplicated UTIs.

E. In patients with particular types of renal stones as well as gout, a low-protein diet may be used. It has no role in patients with UTIs.

---

156. **B.** Cyclic OCPs are the best treatment option for this patient with menorrhagia and dysmenorrhea. Over a period of 6 months, her symptoms should diminish. Eventually, women who cycle on OCPs will have minimal bleeding because of the endometrial atrophy that develops with OCP administration.

A. In the absence of ongoing vaginal bleeding (soaking more than 1 pad per hour), D&C is not indicated.

C, E. Neither GnRH nor progestin therapy is an appropriate treatment option for this patient. GnRH is used in the setting of uterine fibroids, but on this patient's US there are no such masses.

D. Although endometrial ablation would likely stop the patient's bleeding, it would also compromise her future fertility and, therefore, is not the best treatment option.

---

157. **B.** The etiology of this woman's hemorrhage is most likely her submucosal fibroid, shown beginning to prolapse into the vagina. She has already lost enough blood to cause significant symptoms of anemia. While she will likely need definitive treatment in the form of a hysterectomy, she is currently hemodynamically unstable and should first be stabilized with a blood transfusion. Emergent hysterectomy or uterine artery embolization could be performed if bleeding was refractory to hormonal treatment. Once the patient is stable, the fibroid can likely be removed vaginally by grasping it with a toothed tenaculum and twisting. If it is not prolapsed through the cervix, then it can be removed with hysteroscopic resection.

A. Depot Lupron (leuprolide) is a GnRH analog that inhibits gonadotropin release and essentially creates a chemical menopause, causing fibroids to stop growing and possibly shrink in size. At this time, it is not employed as a long-term treatment for fibroids because its prolonged use can lead to bone density loss. Lupron is administered in some women in anticipation of surgery (i.e., hysterectomy) to make surgery safer by decreasing the fibroid bulk and diminishing the potential for blood loss. Patients will often be placed on concurrent iron replacement to increase the hematocrit prior to surgery. While certainly an option for this patient, administration of Lupron is not the most appropriate next step in her treatment.

C. This woman is experiencing symptomatic anemia, making observation an inappropriate option. If she refused blood transfusion, she should be intravenously hydrated at minimum.

D. Hysterectomy would be a definitive treatment in this patient. Before this procedure is performed, however, other causes of bleeding (e.g., endometrial cancer) as well as ovarian and cervical abnormalities (e.g., malignancy) should be evaluated, because such findings could alter the nature of the hysterectomy (e.g., radical hysterectomy versus simple hysterectomy, preservation of ovaries versus bilateral salpingo-oophorectomy).

E. Endometrial ablation is a process in which the endometrial lining is destroyed, usually via thermal means, to stop dysfunctional uterine bleeding. While this method might reduce the patient's bleeding, it would not address the most likely cause of her bleeding (i.e., fibroids).

158. **E.** Placenta previa is the abnormal implantation of the placenta over the cervical os. Depending on how much of the cervix is covered by the placenta, placenta previa is further classified as complete, partial, or marginal. As the lower uterine segment grows, placental attachments can be disrupted, leading to bleeding that ranges from spotting to profuse hemorrhage. One in 200 births is affected by placenta previa, which accounts for 20% of antepartum hemorrhage. Management of placenta previa varies, but most providers will agree that the patient should be placed on pelvic rest (i.e., no intercourse). Bleeding episodes warrant admission for observation to monitor fetal and maternal well-being, and administration of corticosteroids for fetal lung maturity if appropriate (24 to 34 weeks GA).

A. Immediate delivery is warranted only in the event of nonreassuring fetal status, life-threatening hemorrhage, or unstoppable labor. Otherwise, patients are delivered at 36 weeks via cesarean section, usually after confirmation of fetal lung maturity via amniocentesis.

B. Blood transfusion is warranted in situations involving severe blood loss and anemia. Such is not the case in this hemodynamically stable patient.

C. At 33 5/7 weeks GA, fetal lung maturity is unlikely. Thus, if delivery were warranted at this GA, amniocentesis would not be useful.

D. Hormonal management has no role in bleeding in placenta previa, as this kind of bleeding is related to placental detachment rather than endometrial abnormalities.

159. **A.** LGV is caused by the L serotypes of *Chlamydia trachomatis*.

B. The classic LGV lesion is a painless—not painful—papule or shallow ulcer in the genital region that can be transient. This patient has advanced to the inguinal stage.

C. LGV is treated with a 3-week course of doxycycline, which may be repeated if the disease is persistent. Surgical exploration of lymph nodes is not part of therapy.

D. The third stage of LGV, known as anogenital syndrome, involves proctocolitis, rectal stricture, or rectovaginal fistula.

E. LGV is a sexually transmitted infection.

160. **B.** Vaginal wall hematomas can result from injury to a blood vessel in the vaginal wall that does not disrupt the overlying epithelium. They are usually diagnosed while the patient is still hospitalized, as affected patients often experience severe vaginal pain, difficulty walking, or larger than expected drops in hematocrit. However, hematomas that develop slowly can be missed until after discharge, when the patient eventually becomes symptomatic. Management can be expectant unless the hematoma is expanding or tense, in which case it should be evacuated. The wound frequently has to be packed, because bleeding vessels cannot always be identified for ligation.

A. While this is a large drop in hematocrit for a vaginal delivery, the patient is asymptomatic. In the absence of cardiac risk factors, most young, healthy patients can withstand a hematocrit of 22, making the risks of transfusion greater than the benefits in this situation.

C. While iron replacement is warranted, the patient should not be discharged home without evacuation of the hematoma because the hematoma is symptomatic, tense, and possibly expanding. On rare occasions, concealed hemorrhage can be life-threatening if severe. Sitz baths are not appropriate therapy for vaginal/vulvar hematomas.

D. Pitocin has no role in the case of vaginal wall hematoma. It is helpful only in cases involving bleeding due to decreased uterine tone.

E. Uterine artery embolization is not appropriate treatment for a vaginal wall hematoma, because the bleeding is not uterine in origin and such treatment could potentially lead to decreased fertility. The injured vessel and its surrounding vaginal tissue must be addressed.

161. **B.** Condyloma acuminata, or genital warts, are caused by HPV. (Different serotypes of HPV are responsible for cervical cancer.) Genital warts can occur throughout the anogenital region. Treatment regimens vary and include topical medicines, cryotherapy, laser vaporization, and local excision.

A. This patient has pubic lice, or crabs, which are caused by infection with *Phthirus pubis*. Treatment involves application of lindane to affected areas.

C. Chancroid is caused by infection with *Haemophilus ducreyi* and is characterized by a painful ulcer with possible inguinal lymphadenopathy. Diagnosis is made clinically, because *Haemophilus ducreyi* is difficult to culture. Multiple treatment regimens exist, including ceftriaxone 250 mg intramuscularly once; single dose of azithromycin 1 g; or erythromycin 500 mg QID for 7 days.

D. Scabies is caused by infection with the itch mite *Sarcoptes scabiei*. It is similar to infection with pubic lice, but the distribution occurs throughout the body and characteristic burrows can often be identified. Treatment also involves lindane application to affected areas.

E. Syphilis is caused by infection with *Treponema pallidum*. This systemic disease progresses through three stages if left untreated. Primary syphilis is characterized by a painless chancre. Secondary syphilis involves a maculopapular rash, appearing characteristically on the palms and the soles of the feet. Tertiary syphilis is characterized by neurologic manifestations (e.g., tabes dorsalis), aortitis, and gummas (granulomas) of skin and bones. Diagnosis of syphilis is made via nonspecific antibody tests: rapid plasma reagin (RPR) or Venereal Disease Research Laboratory (VDRL). Positive results are confirmed with either the microhemagglutination assay for antibodies to *T. pallidum* (MHATP) or the fluorescent treponemal antibody absorption (FTA-ABS) test. Treatment of early syphilis consists of a one-time dose of 2.4 million units of penicillin G given intramuscularly. This therapy is repeated weekly for 3 weeks in cases of syphilis persisting for longer than 1 year. Because neurosyphilis is more severe, treatment involves 2 to 4 million units of penicillin G every 4 hours for 10 to 14 days.

162. **A.** Wound seromas can result in wound separation when pockets of serosanguineous fluid become trapped beneath the surface of the skin and lead to poor wound healing. Obesity is a risk factor for the development of seromas. Treatment involves exploration of the wound to disrupt any subcutaneous loculations, followed by irrigation and debridement. Finally, the wound should be packed with moist dressings and allowed to close via secondary intention. Dressing changes should be performed twice a day during the healing period, and the patient should be instructed regarding daily wound care.

B. If evidence of a cellulitis (e.g., erythema) was found, oral antibiotics to cover skin flora could be prescribed. Otherwise, the wound needs to heal by secondary intention.

C. While irrigation and debridement are part of care, a wound that has a 3-cm track and is 4 cm deep is unlikely to heal if the overlying skin is merely reapproximated with steristrips. Once the wound has sufficiently healed by secondary intention and is shallow, consideration can be given to steristrip closure.

D. One study of surgical reclosure of disrupted cesarean section wounds as compared to healing by secondary intention showed that wound healing time could be significantly shortened by performing such reclosure. However, all wounds were first managed via irrigation and debridement for a minimum of 4 days before closure was considered. While this is an option for this patient, current practice supports healing by secondary intention.

E. Expectant management is not appropriate in the setting of wound seromas.

163. **E.** A patient who arrives to the hospital with painful contractions and 8 cm dilated is in the active phase of labor, and delivery should be considered imminent. In the absence of prenatal care and with a poor history, it is difficult to assess GA, which is important in terms of preparing and caring for the newborn. Tocolysis at 8-cm dilation is unlikely to be successful as well as unnecessary in this patient, who is probably at term or near to it based on bedside US measurements consistent with a term fetus. Routine prenatal labs as well as a urine toxicology screen should be obtained because the patient did not have prenatal care and to assess for possible substance-induced preterm labor. Otherwise, the patient should be managed like all other laboring patients.

A. Antenatal corticosteroids have been shown to improve fetal outcomes by promoting fetal lung maturity and decreasing the incidence of intraventricular hemorrhages. However, their benefits have been proven only in fetuses who have achieved viability (greater than 24 weeks GA) and in those less than 34 weeks GA, beyond which the incidence of respiratory distress syndrome (RDS) is low (but not insignificant). Additionally, benefit is generally seen only if the fetus is exposed for at least 24 to 48 hours.

B. See the explanation for E.

C. Amniocentesis to assess fetal lung maturity is not appropriate because delivery is imminent.

D. While formal US can estimate fetal age, this patient will likely deliver before she goes for the study. A bedside US for estimated fetal weight and GA can be performed quickly to advise the nursery. Of note, the margin of error in US varies with GA: It can be off by 1 week in the first trimester, 2 weeks in the second trimester, and 3 weeks in the third trimester. Thus this patient could be anywhere between 35 and 41 weeks GA.

---

164. **E.** The diagnosis of preeclampsia is made with three findings: (1) elevation of the BP above 140/90 at least two times, 4 to 6 hours apart; (2) significant proteinuria, exceeding 300 mg in a 24-hour urine collection; and (3) nondependent edema of the face and hands.

A. The CBC helps rule out the diagnosis of severe preeclampsia. A low platelet count can be seen in the setting of HELLP syndrome. Elevation of the hematocrit secondary to hemoconcentration can be seen in preeclampsia, but is not part of the diagnostic criteria.

B, D. Glomerular filtration rate (GFR) and creatinine clearance can be decreased in preeclampsia, resulting in decreased uric acid excretion and elevated serum levels. However, these findings are not part of the diagnostic criteria for preeclampsia. The GFR's only diagnostic use is in patients who have baseline proteinuria and hypertension in whom the diagnosis is difficult to make.

C. Severe preeclampsia can lead to RBC hemolysis, which would elevate lactate dehydrogenase (LDH) levels.

---

165. **C.** This patient has the classic findings of trichomonas, which is caused by infection with *Trichomonas vaginalis*, a unicellular protozoan that is sexually transmitted. Signs and symptoms include profuse, frothy, foul-smelling discharge and a "strawberry" cervix (i.e., erythematous, punctate cervical epithelium). Diagnosis is made by visualization of the motile organisms on wet mount. Treatment consists of a single 2-g dose of metronidazole. Clotrimazole cream for 7 days is another treatment alternative.

A, B. The wet mount does not show the classic clue cells of bacterial vaginosis (BV)—namely, vaginal epithelial cells that are covered with bacteria, thus making the cell's borders appear indistinct. BV is often associated with a fishy-smelling discharge. Treatment for BV includes oral metronidazole 500 mg BID for 7 days or clindamycin 300 mg TID for 7 days. These antibiotics can also be used in gel or cream form intravaginally. Miconazole cream is not an appropriate therapy for bacterial vaginosis.

D. See the explanation for C. Miconazole cream is not an appropriate therapy for trichomonas.

E. Wet mounts for suspected yeast infections should be prepared with potassium hydroxide (KOH) rather than saline to evaluate for the characteristic branching pseudohyphae of *Candida albicans*. Yeast vaginitis typically produces a thick, white, pruritic discharge. Treatment relies on any of the azole creams (e.g., miconazole, terazole) or a single 150-mg dose of oral fluconazole (Diflucan).

---

166. **C.** The adnexal mass identified on the physical and US exams is most likely a TOA, also referred to as a TOC when it is not walled off as in the case of abscesses. TOAs/TOCs typically result from persistent PID and involve the fallopian tube and adjacent ovary. This patient exhibits classic signs and symptoms of pelvic infection (e.g., fever, leukocytosis with left shift, cervical motion tenderness), and the diagnosis is confirmed with US. Blood cultures should be obtained to rule out sepsis. Treatment involves inpatient IV broad-spectrum antibiotics such as cefoxitin and doxycycline or triple antibiotics until 48 hours afebrile, followed by a 10- to 14-day course of oral antibiotics upon her discharge home. If clinical improvement is not achieved with antibiotics, surgical removal (usually via unilateral salpingo-oophorectomy) may be necessary.

A. This patient does not have TSS, which is caused by the toxic shock syndrome toxin-1 (TSST-1) produced by *Staphylococcus aureus*. Historically, TSS has been associated with vaginal infections caused by tampon usage. Signs and symptoms include high fever, hypotension, late-onset desquamation of palms and soles, erythematous rash, and thrombocytopenia. Patients can become very ill, necessitating inpatient management, which consists mostly of supportive care and use of pressors as needed to maintain BP. IV antibiotics have not been shown to decrease the length of acute illness because symptoms are caused by the exotoxin.

B. The adnexal mass in this young patient with symptoms of infection is unlikely to be an ovarian malignancy. She is not having any symptoms of cancer, and imaging studies do not support such a diagnosis (e.g., no omental cake, solid and cystic mass).

D. See the explanation for C. Outpatient management is not appropriate in the acute setting.

E. Endometritis is an intrauterine infection seen most commonly after cesarean section, vaginal delivery, dilation and curettage, and IUD placement. When it involves the myometrium, it is called endomyometritis. While endometritis can present with symptoms similar to those seen with TOAs/TOCs, it is not associated with an adnexal mass. Treatment consists of inpatient IV antibiotics until the patient has been afebrile for 48 hours.

167. | **A.** This patient has some of the classic signs and symptoms of endometriosis: dysmenorrhea, dyspareunia, uterosacral nodularity, likely endometrioma, and infertility. Endometriosis is a chronic condition in which endometrial tissue occurs outside of the uterus (typically on pelvic organs such as the ovary, cul-de-sac, or uterus). Endometriosis implants can become cyclically painful. They can also take the form of endometriomas, known as "chocolate cysts," which are ovarian endometriosis cysts filled with dark, old blood. They are not malignant, but can be painful and are at risk for torsion if large. Endometriosis is associated with infertility, possibly resulting from adhesions, scarring, and alteration of normal pelvic anatomy. Endometriosis can only be truly diagnosed by visualizing endometriosis implants within the pelvis, which is usually achieved via laparoscopy. Implants can be excised or ablated during surgery. OCPs and NSAIDs are appropriate medical treatment for endometriosis. Because this patient is trying to conceive, however, OCPs are not the optimal choice. Of note, because the patient has been trying to conceive for 1 year, an infertility evaluation should be initiated. If this evaluation returns negative, consideration should be given to diagnostic laparoscopy, whereby a diagnosis of endometriosis can be formally made and, if present, implants can be excised or ablated in an attempt to improve fertility.

B. See the explanation for A.

C. Ovarian cancer is rare in a 32-year-old patient. She is not experiencing any concerning symptoms (e.g., early satiety, bloating, weight changes, fatigue). Additionally, the US findings do not support an ovarian malignancy.

D. Mittelschmerz is midcycle pain thought to be due to ovulation. This patient's pain occurs at the start of her cycle.

E. No fibroids are identified on this patient's physical or US exams. Additionally, fibroids do not typically cause pain unless they are degenerating. Note that not all fibroids are managed via hysterectomy, especially in women desiring preservation of fertility.

168. | **D.** The fetus is considered previable until 24 weeks GA. Unfortunately, ROM before viability means the end of the pregnancy. If ROM occurs before the onset of labor, it is called PROM. This case is an example of PPROM (less than 37 weeks GA). At 19 weeks GA, the chance of the pregnancy lasting until viability is slim to none. Once rupture of membranes occurs, the potential for labor and/or infection increases. In fact, it is thought that PPROM occurs as a result of subclinical infection. As such, tocolysis has no role here, as maintenance of an infected pregnancy increases the risk of maternal infection and sepsis. After appropriate counseling and discussion, management of PPROM typically involves termination of the nonviable pregnancy via labor induction. Although expectant management is an option while awaiting onset of spontaneous labor, the risk of infection increases with time so most providers will advocate a more active approach (e.g., labor induction).

A. Corticosteroids are not administered to promote fetal lung maturity unless a fetus is viable.

B. See the explanation for D. Some institutions will administer tocolysis for 48 hours in the absence of signs or symptoms of infection in an effort to administer antenatal corticosteroids to promote fetal lung maturity.

C. While PPROM may result from infection and may subsequently lead to worsening infection, administration of antibiotics is not appropriate in an effort to prolong the pregnancy in the setting of a previable fetus. In the setting of overt infection, administration of antibiotics and labor induction should be initiated as soon as possible.

E. Fetal monitoring is not done on a continuous basis on previable fetuses. Certainly in the case of pregnancy termination, it is not necessary and even cruel to monitor the fetus during labor induction.

---

169. **B.** Colicky back/abdominal pain with CVAT and hematuria are highly suspicious for nephrolithiasis. It is not unusual for patients with nephrolithiasis or other abdominal pain to experience contractions, but these contractions are more consistent with uterine irritability than with labor. Treatment of nephrolithiasis in pregnancy is expectant with IV fluids and pain control. If imaging studies reveal large calculi resulting in significant hydronephrosis or hydroureter, or persistent infection/pyelonephritis, consideration should be given to placement of a nephrostomy tube to drain the kidney.

A. Pregnancy is a contraindication to extracorporeal shock wave lithotripsy (ESWL).

C, D. In the absence of fever, urinalysis consistent with infection, and leukocytosis with left shift, this is unlikely to be a pyelonephritis. Nevertheless, this diagnosis is important to consider because pregnancy does increase urinary stasis both by relaxation of smooth muscle and through compression of ureters by the enlarging uterus. In the event of pyelonephritis, initial treatment of pregnant patients should always be as inpatients with IV antibiotics so that maternal and fetal well-being can be monitored in the early stages.

E. Despite regular contractions, this patient is not dilating her cervix and is therefore not in preterm labor. However, serial cervical exams should be performed at least initially to rule out labor.

---

170. **D.** Magnesium sulfate has been shown to be the most effective agent in preventing recurrent seizures in eclamptic patients. It can also be effective in interrupting the event, and can usually given as a 10-g IM load to patients without an IV placed.

A, C. Until recently, phenytoin represented the drug of choice to prevent recurrent seizures in eclampsia in much of the world. Several studies have since demonstrated magnesium sulfate's efficacy. Like phenytoin, phenobarbital may help to prevent recurrent seizures, but does not seem to be as effective in randomized trials.

B. If the patient is actively seizing, diazepam or another short-acting benzodiazepine is commonly used to break the ongoing seizure activity.

E. The fetal heart rate tracing is currently reassuring. While the patient should be transferred to labor and delivery for labor induction, emergent delivery is unnecessary.

171. **E.** This patient has the classic signs and symptoms of genital herpes and is likely suffering from a primary outbreak, which can often be preceded by a flu-like illness. Herpes is caused by infection with herpes simplex virus (HSV). There are two strains of this virus: HSV-1, which tends to cause oral herpes, and HSV-2, which tends to cause genital outbreaks. However, both types can be found in either region. Because it is a viral infection, herpes can recur after the initial outbreak, with the frequency of recurrences varying between individuals. Diagnosis is usually via visualization of the characteristic cropped vesicles and ulcers, but confirmation can be achieved with viral culture or Tzanck smear to evaluate for multinucleated giant cells. Treatment for herpes relies on acyclovir to shorten the course of the outbreak. People who suffer from frequent recurrences can also take daily acyclovir for suppression therapy. Of note, because lesions can occur throughout the genital area and are transmitted by direct contact, condom usage cannot prevent transmission of herpes.

A. Genital warts are caused by infection with certain serotypes of human papillomavirus (HPV), a sexually transmitted pathogen. Warts, also known as *condyloma acuminata*, are typically painless, raised, and papillomatous or spiky in appearance. Treatment involves excision, cryotherapy, laser ablation, and a variety of topical medications (e.g., trichloroacetic acid, podophyllin, 5-fluorouracil, imiquimod, and podofilox). This patient's lesions are not characteristic of genital warts.

B. Metronidazole is not appropriate therapy for genital warts.

C. *Molluscum contagiosum* is spread via direct contact with an affected area. The infectious organism is a pox virus, which results in the characteristic lesion, a 1- to 5-mm domed papule with an umbilicated center. Lesions are typically painless. Treatment involves expectant management, as lesions generally resolve on their own. Lesions can also be treated with excision, cryotherapy, or application of trichloroacetic acid.

D. This patient does have genital herpes, but hydrocortisone cream is not an appropriate therapy for this STD.

172. **A.** Persistent vaginal bleeding after pregnancy termination is concerning for a complication such as retained POCs, uterine perforation, or cervical laceration. After complete uterine evacuation, the endometrium should appear thin on US. The fact that this patient's endometrial cavity is thick and heterogeneous is suspicious for incomplete uterine evacuation. The most efficient way to stop her bleeding is suction curettage. This procedure can be performed under US guidance to ensure complete uterine evacuation. While the same effect might be achieved with administration of agents that promote uterine tone and contractions (e.g., methergine, misoprostol), incomplete evacuation would necessitate further suction curettage.

B. Expectant management is not appropriate in this patient, who has symptoms consistent with anemia. The uterus will continue to bleed until it is completely evacuated.

C. A thick endometrial complex on US is not normal after D&E.

D. Cervical laceration is not relevant here, as the cervix appears intact on exam. However, because cervical trauma can occur during D&E, it should be considered in the differential diagnosis for persistent vaginal bleeding. Careful exam at the end of the procedure is important.

E. Uterine perforation is a rare but serious complication of D&E. Fortunately, it is unlikely in this patient, who has no GI symptoms, a benign abdomen, and no free fluid on US. Moreover, the patient has an obvious and more common explanation for her persistent bleeding (i.e., retained POCs). If bleeding persists after the uterus is completely evacuated or the patient develops an acute abdomen, consideration should be given to diagnostic laparoscopy to visualize the uterus and possibly repair any damage.

173. **D.** Incompetent cervix entails painless dilation of the cervix occurring in the second trimester. While it should be differentiated from preterm labor, which consists of cervical dilation in response to uterine contractions, this distinction can be difficult to make at times because advanced cervical dilation can lead to contractions, in addition to infection or PROM that can also lead to contractions. Incompetent cervix tends to occur in the second trimester before fetuses reach viability, so it often leads to pregnancy loss. Treatment for pregnancies beyond 24 weeks is similar to treatment for preterm labor: magnesium sulfate tocolysis and administration of corticosteroids for fetal lung maturity. Treatment options vary in previable fetuses depending on the degree of dilation. Most patients with advanced dilation are managed expectantly to see whether labor will ensue. Because of the possibility of delivering a previable neonate at 23 to 25 weeks, termination of pregnancy is offered. An attempt can be made to place an emergent cerclage, which is a permanent suture placed around the cervix at the level of the cervical–vaginal junction (McDonald cerclage) or the internal cervical os (Shirodkar cerclage) in an effort to prevent further dilation. If successful, the cerclage is removed at approximately 36 to 38 weeks in anticipation of spontaneous labor. However, the cerclage should be removed at any time that unstoppable labor occurs (even if it is preterm), as cervical trauma can be sustained if a woman is allowed to labor with a cerclage in place. In this patient who has ROM in addition to an incompetent cervix remote from viability (i.e., 24 weeks GA), the prognosis is grim. Cerclage should not be offered, and termination via either D&E or induction of labor should be strongly encouraged. If the patient wishes expectant management, it should be done only with the understanding that if she develops any signs of infection, termination of pregnancy should proceed at that time.

A. Risk factors for cervical incompetence include uterine anomalies, multiple prior D&E procedures, cervical surgery, and maternal diethylstilbestrol (DES) exposure. Most cases of cervical incompetence happen to women with no identifiable risk factors. Pap smear screening has not been associated with any complications of pregnancy.

B. See the explanation for D.

C. If a patient has experienced a prior delivery/fetal loss due to incompetent cervix, a prophylactic cerclage should be offered in subsequent pregnancies and placed between 12 and 14 weeks GA.

E. Incompetent cervix commonly occurs beyond 17 to 18 weeks of gestation, so a 14-week US would not be a good diagnostic tool for cervical incompetence.

174. **D.** Vulvar cancer is primarily treated with surgical excision with wide margins. Additionally, exploration of lymph nodes is critical. For disease beyond stage I, the contralateral groin lymph nodes should also be evaluated. In poor surgical candidates, such as this patient, as well as in patients with disease recurrences, pelvic radiation can be used to decrease tumor bulk. Prognosis is directly related to the number of lymph nodes involved, with 5-year survival rates as follows: more than 90% with one positive lymph node, 75% to 80% with two positive lymph nodes, and less than 15% with three or more positive lymph nodes.

A. Vulvar cancer is actually quite uncommon, accounting for only 5% of the various gynecologic malignancies. Risk factors include advanced age (average age of diagnosis is sixties), diabetes, hypertension, obesity, low socioeconomic status, and prior vulvar disorders.

B. Symptoms of vulvar cancer tend to be local at the site of the mass. Bleeding, pain, and pruritis are common, but ascites and bloating are not characteristic of vulvar cancer.

C. Some 85% to 90% of vulvar cancer entails squamous cell carcinoma (SCC), which can appear as a fungating mass or an indurated ulcer. It spreads primarily via lymphatics but can also spread via direct extension. Malignant melanoma accounts for 5% to 10% of vulvar cancers. Unlike in SCC, the depth of invasion determines prognosis in melanoma. Basal cell carcinoma accounts for 2% to 3% of vulvar cancers. The remaining 1% comprises very rare types of vulvar cancers (e.g., leiomyosarcomas, fibrous histiocytomas).

E. Vulvar cancer is surgically staged and mere palpation of the lymph nodes is insufficient. In fact, 27% of patients with positive lymph nodes do not have palpable nodes on physical exam. Staging is based on size, extent of spread, and nodal involvement.

175. **C.** Mastitis can be treated by oral antibiotics that will cover maternal skin flora or the infant's oral flora. First-generation cephalosporins or dicloxacillin are commonly used. Admission for IV antibiotics is rarely necessary, and only in cases where oral antibiotics have failed to resolve symptoms or the patient cannot tolerate oral medications.

A. Breast pain due to mastitis can be treated symptomatically with NSAIDs or occasionally with acetaminophen and codeine. There is no reason that acetaminophen needs to be used alone, although in very mild cases it may afford some pain relief.

B. It is important to continue breastfeeding or pumping breast milk during the acute phase of the infection to prevent the intraductal accumulation of infected material. Patients should be reassured that because most cases of mastitis are caused by the patient's skin flora or the infant's oral flora, it is not harmful to continue breastfeeding.

D, E. See the explanation for C.

176. **C.** Adnexal torsion is the twisting of the ovary or adnexa around the ovarian pedicle, resulting in vascular obstruction. Although uncommon, it is an emergency and requires operative intervention. Patients occasionally report prior occurrences of similar pain as the offending cyst or neoplasm enlarges and intermittently undergoes torsion. It can be associated with a mild fever, normal WBC count, nausea, and vomiting. Diagnosis can be confirmed by US, which typically shows an enlarged ovary that is uniformly echogenic with decreased Doppler flow.

A. Although this patient has pain localizing to the RLQ, acute appendicitis generally presents with anorexia, fever, leukocytosis, and, not uncommonly, an acute abdomen. With an identifiable adnexal mass, the etiology of the pain is unlikely to be due to other causes.

B. The patient has a negative pregnancy test.

D. Salpingitis typically presents with fever, elevated WBC count, vaginal discharge, and cervical motion tenderness.

E. Although certainly more common than adnexal torsion, ruptured ovarian cysts typically produce pain that is bilateral and begins at or after ovulation. If this case truly involved rupture of an ovarian cyst, the patient would usually experience more diffuse pelvic pain. Also, the patient might have presented with a decreased hematocrit if bleeding were severe. US would show free fluid in the cul-de-sac and is less likely than torsion to reveal the presence of an enlarged adnexal mass.

177. **D.** In an inevitable abortion, the patient will experience vaginal bleeding and a dilated cervix in a pregnancy less than 20 weeks GA but no expulsion of POCs. Although the use of prostaglandins to promote the expulsion of the POCs is an option, D&C is preferential in the setting of heavy bleeding. Expectant management is also an option for patients not anxious about bleeding and cramping at home. Of note, if this patient were Rh D (−), RhoGAM administration would be necessary to prevent alloimmunization in subsequent pregnancies.

A. In any pregnant woman presenting with vaginal bleeding and abdominal pain, ectopic pregnancy must be ruled out. The presence of an intrauterine gestational sac makes the likelihood of a concurrent extrauterine pregnancy highly unlikely, but ectopic pregnancy must still be excluded by history, physical exam, labs, and a careful survey of the lower pelvis by US.

B. A threatened abortion is defined by vaginal bleeding in a pregnancy less than 20 weeks GA in the presence of a closed cervical os and no expulsion of POCs. In the setting of a desired pregnancy, the patient should be given instructions for pelvic rest and followed for continued bleeding rather than proceed prematurely to definitive procedures such as D&C.

C. An incomplete abortion involves the partial expulsion of POCs prior to 20 weeks gestation. It can be allowed to complete on its own, or the patient can be offered D&C or D&E.

E. A complete abortion involves the complete expulsion of all POCs prior to 20 weeks gestation. Patients should be followed for signs of infection and recurrent bleeding.

178. | **C.** Outpatient treatment of uncomplicated PID has been promoted over the past decade. To qualify for this treatment, the patient must have no signs of pelvic abscess (adnexal masses or abscesses seen on US) or perihepatitis (liver transaminase elevations or RUQ tenderness). Furthermore, patients must be nonpregnant and reliable. Severely ill patients not tolerating oral intake are unlikely to comply with medication regimens and will need hospitalization for parenteral therapy.

A, B. Because untreated PID can lead to infertility, hospitalization is generally recommended but not required for reproductive-age patients. Conversely, it is highly recommended that adolescents or any patients in whom compliance may be an issue be hospitalized for treatment.

D. Adnexal tenderness is part of the diagnostic criteria of PID, and is not particularly an indication for hospitalization.

E. Patients with a penicillin allergy can either be treated without penicillins and cephalosporins, or be treated with a cephalosporin in the ED with the knowledge that there is only a 10% to 15% cross-allergic response. In patients with a history of anaphylaxis to penicillin, adequate coverage can be obtained with oral levofloxacin and clindamycin.

179. | **E.** This patient is diagnosed with a ruptured ectopic pregnancy based on the fact that she has no identifiable intrauterine pregnancy at a GA where one should easily be found by US. Additionally, she has free fluid in the cul-de-sac suggestive of rupture and a history of PID, which is a known risk factor for ectopic pregnancy. The decision to take the patient emergently to the operating room is based on the high probability for a ruptured ectopic pregnancy and the fact that the patient has an acute abdomen and appears hemodynamically unstable.

A, B. Uterine curettage or culdocentesis is unnecessary as the diagnosis is highly likely given the US findings.

C, D. Although serial quantitative β-hCG levels would have been helpful in diagnosis prior to rupture, obtaining a value now does not affect the patient's management. Medical management is not appropriate once the ectopic pregnancy has ruptured.

180. | **B.** The patient should be treated empirically for chlamydia and gonorrhea. Azithromycin 1 g PO covers *Chlamydia trachomatis*, and ceftriaxone 250 mg IM covers *Neisseria gonorrhoea*.

A. Simple initiation of OCPs at this time will not ensure pregnancy prevention. Instead, the patient should be tested for preexisting pregnancy and offered emergency contraception. If she does not have menses within 21 days, she is advised to see her gynecologist for follow-up.

C. Even if the patient objects to having this crime reported, it is nevertheless a reportable crime. Often, the nursing staff in the ED will already have done so, but it is important that the physician seeing the patient follows up and makes sure that the crime has been reported. Along these lines, evidence of the crime needs to be collected as well. The patient can then decide whether to give a report to the police once they become involved.

D, E. Despite no initial visual evidence of sperm on a wet prep slide, it is still possible that intravaginal ejaculation did occur. As a consequence, the patient should be offered emergency contraception, baseline HIV testing, and AZT prophylaxis.

---

181. **D.** This patient has a presentation that is worrisome for TSS, which carries a high mortality rate; all patients with this condition should be hospitalized. In severe cases, pressors may be required to stabilize BPs. With aggressive supportive management, it is likely that mortality can be reduced.

A. TSS is caused by *Staphylococcus aureus* exotoxin. Its systemic absorption leads to fever, rash, and desquamation of palms and soles.

B. No data exist that support an association between PCOS and TSS. The other potential causes provide portals of entry for infection. One of the most commonly associated findings with TSS is a highly absorbent tampon.

C. Because the exotoxin is absorbed through the vaginal wall, blood cultures are usually negative.

E. Fewer than 300 cases of TSS have been reported annually since 1984.

---

182. **B.** Although the fetal heart tracing (FHT) is not reassuring because it is nonreactive, there is no evidence of acute fetal insult (FHT decelerations or absent variability) that would necessitate emergent delivery at this time. Attempts should be made to achieve reassuring fetal testing by alternative means—for example, by using vibroacoustic stimulation (VAS) to achieve a reactive tracing or by using US to obtain a biophysical profile (BPP). Another method that is used in labor to obtain fetal response as measured by fetal heart rate acceleration is the fetal scalp stimulation.

A. Although elevated, the patient's glucose level does not warrant administration of additional insulin at this time. There is no reason to react to a blood sugar less than 200 in this setting.

C. Assuming the GA is accurate, there is no evidence of fetal benefit from administration of betamethasone beyond 34 weeks GA.

D, E. Delivery is not indicated in this patient unless the FHT becomes nonreassuring. If that were the case, the decision regarding route of delivery would depend on the severity of the nonreassuring FHT as well as fetal presentation. If induction of labor were indicated rather than emergent cesarean section, a prostaglandin agent would be appropriate in this patient with an unfavorable cervix.

---

183. **D.** Because of her history of manual placenta extraction, this patient is at increased risk for development of endomyometritis, which is a polymicrobial infection of the uterine lining and wall. Diagnosis is made by the presence of fever, uterine tenderness, and elevated WBC count. Treatment consists of broad-spectrum antibiotics. D&C is indicated only if retained POCs is suspected, which is not the case in this patient whose lochia has decreased appropriately.

A. Given her history of decreased vaginal bleeding, stable vital signs, and hematocrit, this patient does not have a delayed postpartum hemorrhage.

B. Placenta accreta (abnormal adherence of the placenta to the uterine wall) would be manifested as continued vaginal bleeding unresponsive to contractile agents and is more likely to be diagnosed immediately postpartum rather than 1 week later.

C. The patient shows no evidence of a vaginal hematoma, which occurs when the trauma of delivery injures a blood vessel without disrupting the overlying epithelium. Such hematomas can be managed expectantly, unless the patient is hemodynamically unstable, in which case surgical exploration and ligation of the disrupted vessel(s) may be required.

E. See the explanation for D.

184. **B.** A lesion that is confined to the cervix, more than 5 mm invasive, and less than 4 cm wide is a stage Ib1 lesion. Approximately 40% of cervical cancer is stage Ib at diagnosis; cancer at this stage has an 85% cure rate regardless of whether radical hysterectomy or radiation therapy is used. For bulky stage Ib to IVa disease, primary treatment with cisplatin-based chemotherapy in conjunction with radiation therapy can prolong disease-free survival when compared to radiation therapy alone.

A. This is stage Ib1 disease; cone biopsy is appropriate only in microinvasive disease (stages Ia1 and Ia2).

C. Stage Ib2 lesions are more than 4 cm wide.

D, E. Stage II lesions extend beyond the cervix but not to the sidewall, with vaginal involvement in the upper two thirds only. Stage IIa lesions do not involve the parametria, whereas stage IIb lesions have obvious parametrial involvement. Radical hysterectomy is beneficial treatment only for stage IIa or earlier disease. Radiation therapy is indicated once the cancer has spread to the parametria or beyond (stage IIb or later). Primary chemotherapy can be beneficial for both stage IIa and IIb disease.

185. **E.** This patient is most likely having a placental abruption secondary to her elevated BPs and possible preeclampsia. Although the patient is hemodynamically stable and the fetus is premature, emergent delivery by cesarean section is indicated because of nonreassuring fetal status. It is reasonable to check the fetal heart rate in the OR to verify that it is still decreased; such a finding will help determine the rapidity with which the delivery needs to occur.

A. This patient may require blood transfusion because the volume of blood loss in a placental abruption is often underestimated due to concealed bleeding. However, this is not the most appropriate next step given the nonreassuring FHT.

B. Although the fetus is premature and would likely benefit from the administration of betamethasone, immediate delivery is indicated. Thus there would not be sufficient time to benefit from corticosteroids.

C. The use of tocolytics to prolong the pregnancy until fetal lung maturity can be achieved might be indicated in a stable abruption, which is not the case here. If the patient is having a tetanic contraction, it is reasonable to give terbutaline 0.25 mg SQ to promote uterine relaxation.

D. Induction of labor is inappropriate because emergent delivery is indicated.

186. **B. In this patient with a pulmonary embolus who is 24 hours status post an abdominal surgery, IV heparin is the best initial management because it has a short half-life, leads to rapid anticoagulation, can be stopped immediately, and can be reversed with protamine sulfate.**

A. Supplemental oxygen should be provided, but it should not be the only treatment administered to the patient—she will also require medical therapy. Patients who require supplemental oxygen because of shunting should usually be placed on it by means of a nonrebreather face mask. Many patients on nasal cannula will simply breathe through their mouth, decreasing the efficacy of such treatment.

C. Treatment of an acute DVT or PE is now often accomplished with low-molecular-weight heparin. If this patient had delivered vaginally or was a few more days out from her delivery, this therapy would be a reasonable option (see the explanation for B).

D. Eventually, this patient can be converted to warfarin therapy. However, this agent is not a good initial treatment because it often takes several days of therapy to achieve adequate anticoagulation.

E. Furosemide (Lasix) is commonly used in patients with pulmonary edema to facilitate diuresis. It has no role in this patient.

187. **E. Based on her history and physical, the patient has a small bowel obstruction (SBO). Her abdominal X-rays confirm this fact and are further worrisome for bowel perforation with evidence of free air. This patient needs IVs placed for rehydration and immediate exploration in the OR. She should be asked to give informed consent for possible bowel resection, ileostomy, and/or colostomy.**

A. In patients with SBO who are stable, NGT placement and NPO are reasonable plans for management.

B. Although this patient may require TPN at a later time, she has an SBO that has likely perforated and requires emergent laparotomy prior to management of her malnutrition.

C. Laparoscopy is now being utilized for second-look operations for confirmation of absent disease in ovarian cancer. This possibility is not the issue in this patient.

D. In a patient with appendicitis or cholecystitis, this approach is sometimes taken. However, this patient has a perforated viscous and needs to go to the OR immediately.

188. **B. Because continuous OCPs have proven to be effective for this patient, she should be restarted on them. The patient should be informed that she can withdraw from the OCPs approximately twice a year and that it is acceptable to not have regular menses given the cyclical nature of endometriosis pain.**

A. This regimen has proven to be ineffective for the patient in the past, and there is no reason to believe that resuming it now would provide pain relief for her.

C. Although menstrual suppression by progestin treatment (usually medroxyprogesterone depot injection) is effective treatment for some women with endometriosis, it is preferable to resume an effective treatment rather than experiment with new regimens in this patient.

D. GnRH agonists are effective in treating chronic endometriosis pain in 75% to 90% of women. However, their use is generally limited to 6 months due to the side effects associated with estrogen deficiency (bone loss and vasomotor symptoms). Although "add back" regimens have been utilized successfully to counter these side effects, their effectiveness is tempered by the inconvenience and cost of taking additional medications.

E. There is no indication for operative treatment in this patient with endometriosis responsive to medical treatment and no desire for future fertility.

189. **D.** The goals of management in patients with severe hyperemesis gravidarum include maintenance of hydration and nutritional status, as well as symptom relief. Achievement of these goals requires a team approach and often includes consultation with social work and nutrition services. Although many patients will respond to IV hydration and antiemetics, a small percentage may require prolonged hospitalization. If oral intake cannot be tolerated in this setting, it is reasonable to place a pediatric feeding tube, which is usually well tolerated. TPN should be considered only after attempting every other form of nutrition and hydration.

A. Hospitalization will be required if the patient cannot tolerate oral intake.

B. Many patients with hyperemesis gravidarum are conflicted about the pregnancy. A social services consult can provide the added social support they may need.

C. Zofran has been used in pregnancy in these patients for several years with no known teratogenic effects. It is commonly reserved for nausea and vomiting refractory to other first-line antiemetic agents.

E. If the patient cannot tolerate oral intake, a feeding tube should be placed. The feeding tube's tip should be placed in the duodenum, making the feeds more easily tolerated. This is the preferred method of feeding over TPN.

190. **E.** The patient is experiencing dysmenorrhea secondary to outflow obstruction. She has cervical stenosis, which is a known complication of LEEP and other cervical surgeries. The most appropriate treatment for her is cervical dilation, as OCPs will merely decrease the amount of her menstrual flow but will not eliminate the underlying problem. Unfortunately, many patients with cervical stenosis will experience recurrences of the disorder, requiring repeat cervical dilations.

A. Although the patient has a history of instrumentation, she does not have any evidence of infection, making pelvic abscess an unlikely etiology for her symptoms.

B. Although dysmenorrhea is a common symptom of endometriosis, the rest of the patient's history is inconsistent with such a diagnosis, which can only be truly made by diagnostic laparoscopy.

C. Given the typically slow progression of cervical cancer, it is highly unlikely that the patient would develop cervical cancer after being diagnosed with cervical dysplasia and undergoing LEEP only 6 months ago. Additionally, cervical cancer often presents as painless postcoital vaginal bleeding rather than dysmenorrhea.

D. See the explanation for E.

---

191. **A.** Complete moles result from the fertilization of an empty ovum by a normal sperm, which is then thought to duplicate itself. Thus the most common karyotype for complete moles is 46,XX. A partial mole is the fertilization of an ovum with two sperm; its most common karyotype is 69,XXY.

B, C, D. Treatment of complete moles involves immediate suction evacuation of the uterus and gentle curettage. They cannot be managed expectantly, and a hysterectomy would be too extreme. Chemotherapy is indicated only if malignant transformation occurs, which is confirmed by persistently elevated β-hCG levels after uterine evacuation.

E. The risk of developing GTD in subsequent pregnancies is only 5%.

---

192. **D.** This patient is experiencing urinary retention. Given her recent history of urogynecological surgery, the likely etiology is overcorrection of her urinary incontinence with resultant urinary outflow obstruction. The appropriate treatment is placement of a Foley catheter to relieve the obstruction. Surgical exploration and repair are not indicated at this time.

A, B, C. Although the patient's urine sample was not an ideal specimen, the lack of leukocyte esterase and nitrites on urine dipstick makes the diagnosis of UTI unlikely. If clinical suspicion for infection is high, the urine should be cultured. A straight catheter specimen is not necessary, and a single catheterization will not correct this patient's problem. However, once the Foley catheter is placed, antibiotic suppression against UTIs can be considered.

E. The patient may eventually need a repeat surgery to relax the suspension of the bladder neck. This procedure should not happen immediately, nor should it occur without another trial of voiding.

---

193. **B.** Quantitative serum β-hCG will help indicate the most likely diagnosis: molar pregnancy. This patient presents with marked proteinuria and hypertension in the late first trimester. Most preeclampsia is not seen before 20 weeks (and usually not until the third trimester), except in the setting of molar pregnancy. Epigastric pain and severe nausea should also prompt consideration of gastroenteritis, cholestatic disease, pancreatic disease, and hepatitis. However, this patient is afebrile, has normal GI lab values, and proteinuria, moving molar pregnancy to the top of the differential diagnosis. Molar pregnancies have elevated hCG, with levels occasionally exceeding 1 million. The diagnosis will be confirmed by an US that reveals an enlarged uterus filled with hydropic trophoblastic tissue (complete mole) or a fetus with a thickened, hydropic placenta (incomplete mole).

A. CA-125 is a nonspecific tumor marker expressed in many ovarian neoplasms. Ovarian cancer typically presents with vague abdominal complaints, not the acute presentation described here.

C. Serum magnesium levels will not be useful in diagnosing this patient. If she does have preeclampsia secondary to a molar pregnancy, magnesium therapy may be used for seizure prophylaxis.

D. Maternal serum alpha-fetoprotein is, in fact, lower than expected based on GA in molar pregnancies. This finding is not very specific, however; it can result from overestimated GA, chromosomal abnormalities such as trisomies 18 and 21, or maternal obesity. Elevated serum β-hCG is a far more useful diagnostic test in this case.

E. Serum thyroxine is often elevated in molar pregnancy, due to the structural homology of hCG and thyrotropin (thyroid-stimulating hormone, or TSH). Clinical hyperthyroidism is rare, however, and this value, while useful, is not beneficial in the diagnosis of this patient. It would be essential information in the medical and surgical management of this patient.

194. E. The most likely diagnosis is incomplete (partial) molar pregnancy, which results when a normal ovum is fertilized by two sperm. The karyotype is typically triploid, most commonly (80%) 69,XXY. An incomplete mole is more likely because of the presence of embryonic tissue.

A. 46,XX is the most common karyotype for a complete mole, which forms when an empty ovum is fertilized by one sperm. No embryonic/fetal tissue is present. All chromosomes are paternally derived. (46,XX is, of course, the karyotype for a normal female.)

B, C, D. 47,XXY, 47,XX+18, and 47,XX+21 are the karyotypes for Klinefelter's, Edward's, and Down syndromes, respectively. These aneuploidies all increase rates of spontaneous abortion, but the elevated β-hCG level, when combined with the vesicles seen on exam and characteristic sonographic findings, make gestational trophoblastic disease the likely diagnosis. Elevated maternal serum β-hCG is seen in trisomy 21, but not to the level observed in this patient.

195. C. This patient likely has endometriosis, which can be definitively diagnosed only by direct visualization (e.g., diagnostic laparoscopy). Endometriosis is the presence of endometrial cells outside of the endometrial cavity. Several theories have been promulgated regarding the origin of endometriosis. The Halban theory proposes that endometrial cells travel through the lymphatic system to different sites in the pelvis, where they then cause symptoms. Meyer's theory purports that multipotential cells in the peritoneum undergo metaplastic transformation into working endometrium. Sampson theorizes that retrograde menstruation of endometrial cells through the fallopian tubes results in pelvic implants and the symptoms of endometriosis. Endometrial implants can appear as powder-burn, mulberry, or blueberry lesions anywhere in the pelvis. Occasionally, an inverse relationship exists between the amount of disease present and the severity of symptoms.

A. A corpus luteum cyst results from the rupture of the ovarian follicle that resulted in ovulation. It is extremely rare to have bilateral corpus luteum cysts.

B. Scant powder-burn lesions may be present with endometriosis, but the etiology of this patient's pain is most likely due to her sizable bilateral masses, which are probably blood-filled endometriomas, giving the low-attenuation appearance on US.

D. Peritoneal tuberculosis is an extrapulmonary manifestation of tuberculosis characterized by abdominal pain, fever, weight loss, and ascites. It is the leading cause of infertility worldwide, but it is an unlikely source of this patient's cysts and adnexal pain.

E. TOA would be suspected in a patient with cervical motion, uterine, and adnexal tenderness. TOAs are often associated with fever and risk factors for STDs.

196. C. Gonococcal (GC) infections are transmitted at the time of delivery and can cause disseminated illness in the neonate. There is also a theoretical concern that they can cause ascending infections in pregnancy, leading to higher rates of preterm labor and delivery. For this reason, GC infections are treated aggressively in pregnancy.

A. Transmission of toxoplasmosis is most common during the third trimester, but the neonatal complications tend to be milder than those seen with early-pregnancy transmission.

B. HIV transmission can occur transplacentally, but this virus is transmitted more commonly during birth from exposure to blood and vaginal secretions.

D. Varicella zoster virus (VZV) can cause both spontaneous abortions and a fetal infection that can lead to neurologic disease and cutaneous lesions. Patients who are not VZV immune should avoid exposure during pregnancy. If exposed, they should be given immunoglobulin prophylaxis, or VZIG, to decrease the chances of becoming infected.

E. Parvovirus B-19 causes fifth disease in children and occasionally adults. In the fetus, it can lead to myelosuppression, manifested by anemia and fetal hydrops.

197. A. Mittelschmerz (from German; literally, "middle pain") is pain due to the rupture of an ovarian follicle during ovulation, resulting in intraperitoneal fluid or blood that can produce localized or diffuse abdominal pain. The easiest way to prevent future bouts of mittelschmerz is to place the patient on OCPs to suppress ovulation.

B. PID is most commonly seen in young sexually active women with multiple partners. In addition to being in a long-term monogamous relationship, this patient is unlikely to have PID because she is afebrile, has a normal WBC count, and exhibits no cervical motion tenderness or vaginal discharge.

C. Mittelschmerz can frequently be confused with adnexal torsion. The timing and nature of the symptoms in this patient make mittelschmerz a more likely diagnosis. One would expect a more protracted course with adnexal torsion, usually with concomitant nausea and vomiting. A pelvic US might be helpful in the evaluation if the clinical picture were more confusing.

D. The patient has a negative pregnancy test.

E. Left-side pain can occur uncommonly in acute appendicitis. This patient does not have other signs or symptoms that are consistent with appendicitis.

198. **A.** Although numerous risk factors exist for preterm delivery, the biggest risk factor is history of a prior preterm delivery. Other risk factors for preterm labor include multiple gestations, polyhydramnios, being African American, bacterial vaginosis, uterine anomalies, PROM, preeclampsia, and some maternal medical conditions.

B. While it has been theorized that multiple TABs increase the risk of incompetent cervix, no studies to date have correlated history of one prior TAB with preterm delivery.

C. Bacterial vaginosis has been associated with preterm labor, but no such association exists with vaginal candidiasis.

D. A prepregnancy weight of less than 50 kg is a risk factor for preterm delivery, but no such association exists with obesity.

E. While it is true that maternal age less than 20 is associated with preterm delivery, it is not this patient's biggest risk factor.

199. **B.** This patient has a mild case of OHSS, a rare but potentially life-threatening complication of ovulation induction with gonadotropins. In addition to ovarian enlargement, affected patients experience weight gain and abdominal distention. In severe cases, patients can present with ascites, pleural effusion, electrolyte imbalance, hypovolemia, and oliguria. The syndrome is managed by hospitalization, discontinuing gonadotropins, correcting fluid and electrolyte imbalances, and supportive therapy.

A. While adnexal torsion is relatively common in OHSS, this patient's exam and history are not consistent with such a diagnosis. With a diagnosis of adnexal torsion, one would expect nausea, vomiting, and a more concerning pelvic exam.

C. Ectopic pregnancy should be considered in the differential diagnosis of any sexually active woman of child-bearing age who presents with lower abdominal pain. However, the negative pregnancy test and large ovarian mass on US exam make such a diagnosis unlikely. Because the possibility of an early ectopic pregnancy exists, a quantitative β-hCG would assist in confirming the diagnosis.

D. While the patient may have an endometrioma in the pelvis, her acute symptoms and history are more consistent with OHSS.

E. The patient's history of an occluded left fallopian tube might make the diagnosis of PID more likely. However, with the exception of abdominal pain, she has no physical signs or symptoms of PID.

200. | **C.** With a sure LMP and an US showing a smaller than expected gestational sac without cardiac motion, this patient is most likely starting a spontaneous abortion of a nonviable pregnancy. Misoprostol is a prostaglandin that can be administered vaginally or orally to induce cervical dilation and uterine contractions to empty the uterus. It is used for labor induction both at term and in the setting of intrauterine fetal demise. Various protocols exist for its use in early miscarriage in women who do not wish to wait for miscarriage to occur spontaneously (expectant management) or who wish to avoid instrumentation (i.e., D&C).

A. With a closed cervix and a nonviable intrauterine pregnancy (no cardiac motion at a GA when it would certainly be expected), this patient has experienced a missed abortion. If cardiac motion was detected in the setting of vaginal bleeding and cramping but no cervical dilation, this case would be considered a threatened abortion. If the cervix was dilated, and particularly if tissue was present in the cervical os, it would be considered an inevitable abortion. A complete abortion refers to a situation in which a previously pregnant patient has already passed all the pregnancy tissue from the uterus such that the uterus appears empty on US.

B. See the explanation for C.

D. Generally, any pregnant woman who experiences vaginal bleeding should have the blood type and Rh checked so that RhoGAM can be administered if she is Rh negative. RhoGAM should be considered even if the amount of vaginal bleeding is small, because the risks and consequences of Rh isoimmunization can be quite serious while the risks of RhoGAM administration are minimal (e.g., allergic reaction). While this patient is likely to eventually experience vaginal bleeding as the pregnancy spontaneously aborts or she undergoes a medical or surgical evacuation, she currently has not had any vaginal bleeding. Thus RhoGAM is not indicated at this time.

E. In general, recurrent pregnancy loss is not diagnosed or evaluated until after three consecutive abortions. In women of advanced maternal age (AMA, 35 years or older), evaluations may sometimes commence after two consecutive abortions. However, this patient is not considered to be of AMA.

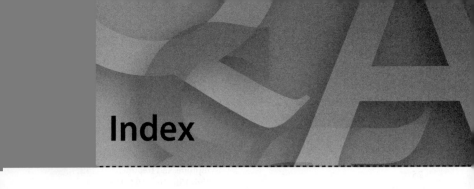

Index

Index note: page references with an *f* or a *t* indicate a figure or table on designated page; page references in **bold** indicate discussion of the subject in the Answers and Explanations sections.